NEURODEGENERATIVE DISEASES - LABORATORY AND CLINICAL RESEARCH

PARKINSONISM

ETIOLOGIES, DIAGNOSIS AND MEDICAL MANAGEMENT

NEURODEGENERATIVE DISEASES - LABORATORY AND CLINICAL RESEARCH

Additional books in this series can be found on Nova's website under the Series tab.

Additional e-books in this series can be found on Nova's website under the e-book tab.

NEURODEGENERATIVE DISEASES - LABORATORY AND CLINICAL RESEARCH

PARKINSONISM

ETIOLOGIES, DIAGNOSIS AND MEDICAL MANAGEMENT

CYNTHIA FISHER
EDITOR

New York

NOTICE TO THE READER

Library of Congress Cataloging-in-Publication Data

Library of Congress Control Number: 2015952553

ISBN: 978-1-63483-865-8

Published by Nova Science Publishers, Inc. † New York

CONTENTS

PREFACE

Parkinson's disease, a common neurologic disorder of dopamine dysfunction, is characterized by motor, cognitive, psychiatric and autonomic symptoms. Parkinsonism has been defined as a complex syndrome with many etiologies. It is most common in the elderly, its cause is unknown and it is represented by idiopathic Parkinson's disease and other neurodegenerative conditions. Chapter one of this book discusses vascular Parkinsonism, which is a type of a Parkinsonism secondary to cerebrovascular disease. Chapter two presents a single blind randomized phase II study comparing surgical intervention with adjustable ventriculo-peritoneal shunt plus dopamine oral therapy versus surgical operation alone in patients affected by idiopathic normal pressure hydrocephalus associated with Parkinsonism. Chapter three reviews the current knowledge regarding the role of Mavridis' atrophy (the parkinsonism-related shrinkage of the human nucleus accumbens) in Parkinson's disease.

Chapter 1 - Parkinsonism has been defined as a complex syndrome with many etiologies. Parkinsonism is most common in the elderly, its cause is unknown and it is represented by idiopathic Parkinson's disease (PD) and other neurodegenerative conditions. PD is the most common cause of parkinsonism and accounts for about 75% of all cases. Vascular parkinsonism (VP) is a type of a parkinsonism secondary to cerebrovascular disease. In population and clinical cohort studies, it accounts for 2.5-12% of all cases of parkinsonism. When the diagnosis includes pathological and imaging studies, VP accounts for 3-6% of all cases of parkinsonism. In a clinico-radiological study of patients with stroke who had deep cerebral infarctions and white matter lesions, it was observed that nearly a third of the patients had one or more parkinsonian signs one year after their stroke.

Edouard Brissaud suggested that Parkinson's disease was due to a lesion in the substantia nigra. In 1929, Critchley made the first description of a type of parkinsonism in elderly patients with high blood pressure caused by cerebrovascular disease, which he called atherosclerotic parkinsonism. He described the course of the disease in these patients as rapid and as preferably affecting the lower limbs, suggesting that multiple vascular lesions in the basal ganglia were presumably responsible for producing the cardinal symptoms in this syndrome. He classified it into five subtypes: 1) parkinsonian symptoms and short-stepping gait; 2) parkinsonism associated with pseudobulbar palsy; 3) parkinsonism with dementia; 4) parkinsonism with pyramidal tract signs; and 5) parkinsonism with cerebellar ataxia. The concept was accepted for decades, until it became controversial, because of the imprecision of its limits, the lack of pathological evidence and because it included heterogeneous conditions. Schwalb and England rejected the concept, arguing that the evidence of vascular change found in some patients with PD could be an incidental finding. Afterwards, Critchley revised his initial concept and introduced the term "vascular pseudo-parkinsonism" to provide it with a broader meaning to vascular participation and to differentiate it from idiopathic PD.

The concept of VP continues to be discussed because of the absence of diagnostic criteria and because of the difficulty that there is, in some cases, in differentiating VP from PD. In addition, the patients included in the initial studies do not meet current criteria for Parkinson's disease. As a rule, however, there is an agreement to replace the term atherosclerotic by vascular because it would thus include ischemic or hemorrhagic lesions not caused by atherosclerosis.

The clinical presentation and background of cardiovascular disease (CVD) may be imprecise. Vascular lesions are frequently found in pathologically confirmed PD(7). The diagnosis of VP is especially complex if we consider that, in elderly patients without parkinsonism, infarcts are frequently found in subcortical cerebral white matter and basal ganglia.

In patients with VP, brain imaging studies are useful for two purposes: to exclude other causes of degenerative parkinsonism (progressive supranuclear palsy) and to discard secondary causes (tumors, hydrocephalus). Computerized tomography (CT) and magnetic resonance imaging (MRI) have contributed to the concept of VP over the past few decades. The presence of cerebrovascular lesions in basal ganglia or subcortical white matter in patients with parkinsonism suggests VP, although this does not exclude a diagnosis of PD.

Because of its broad spectrum, the clinical diagnosis of VP is complex. The definitive diagnosis of VP is neuropathological, although this is not specific because the changes found are those characteristic of small vessel disease and that is why there are doubts about whether VP should be identified as a clinical entity or as a clinical expression of small vessel disease or of an acute focal ischemic lesion.

Chapter 2 - Objective: Idiopathic normal pressure hydrocephalus (iNPH) patients may present, besides the classic triad of symptoms, extrapiramidal parkinsonian like movement disorders. The authors present a single blind randomized phase II study comparing surgical intervention with adjustable ventriculo-peritoneal (VP) shunt plus dopamine oral therapy (group A) versus surgical operation alone (group B) in patients affected by iNPH associated with parkinsonism.

Methods: A detailed screening process included neurological, neurosurgical and neuropsychological evaluations, followed by cerebrospinal fluid (CSF) tap test (TT), resistance outflow (Ro) measurement and CSF neurodegenerative proteins dosage. Outcome was evaluated through the Japanese NPH grading scale-revised (JNPHGSR) and the third section of the Unified Parkinson's Disease Rating Scale (UPDRS).

Results: 54 patients were screened in 36 months; 32/54 (59%) patients (mean age 73.2, range 61-80) met the inclusion criteria, but only 30 were enrolled in the study, since two patients refused to undergo surgery. 15 patients were randomized in group A and 15 in group B. Preoperative 123I-Ioflupane-cerebral SPECT (DaTSCAN) revealed some striatal dopaminergic deficit in 14/30 patients (46.5%). At the final scheduled 12 months follow-up, 23/30 patients (77% overall, 13 from group A and 10 from group B) showed an improvement of the JNPHGRS score; 19/30 patients (63% overall), 12/15 patients of group A (80%) and 7/15 patients of group B (47%), showed an improvement greater than 30% in the motor UPDRS score.

Conclusion: An association between iNPH and parkinsonism may be present in more than half of patients. In these cases, patients may benefit from VP shunt plus dopamine oral therapy.

Chapter 3 - Parkinson's disease (PD), a common neurologic disorder of dopamine (DA) dysfunction, is characterized by motor, cognitive, psychiatric and autonomic symptoms. The nucleus accumbens (NA), a major part of the ventral striatum, belongs to the basal ganglia of the brain. It acts as a limbic-motor interface and plays an important role in motivation and emotional processes. It is the most important pleasure center of the human brain and is involved in some of the most disabling neuropsychiatric disorders, such as PD.

More specifically, the NA is crucially involved in PD, not only in its pathogenesis and clinical manifestations but in the effects of several treatment efforts as well. Mavridis' atrophy (MA) is called the parkinsonism-related shrinkage of the human NA. The purpose of this chapter is to review the current knowledge regarding the role of MA in PD. MA was recently described as a novel research (neuroimaging) finding and there are subsequent important clinical studies confirming this finding. MA is part of the degeneration of the DAergic nigrostriatal system that occurs in PD and this also explains the fact that MA precedes clinical phenotype. Thus, neuronal loss is probably the major cause of MA and, interestingly, degeneration of limbic areas is considered as a pathological consequence of MA. Functional NA changes also accompany MA. It has been shown that MA begins in early-stage PD patients and is correlated with psychiatric symptoms that occur in PD, mainly apathy and impulsive behavior. Moreover, MA is also associated with cognitive PD symptoms. Given that some motor and psychiatric symptoms may share a common pathophysiological process mediated by the NA, the clinical effects of MA are expected to include, apart from neuropsychiatric symptoms, motor symptoms as well; a hypothesis, however, that remains to be confirmed. MA, as an imaging finding, could be used as a risk factor for the expression and/or severity of specific symptoms, such as psychiatric manifestations, in PD patients. Further research is mandatory to enrich our knowledge and improve our understanding of the significance of the role of the MA phenomenon in PD. Future research efforts should focus on the underlying mechanisms of MA, its pathological features, as well as the clinical applications of this imaging finding.

In: Parkinsonism
Editor: Cynthia Fisher

ISBN: 978-1-63483-865-8

Chapter 1

VASCULAR PARKINSONISM: NEW APPROACH

Fernando Alarcón*, MD
Chief of Neurology Department, Professor of Neurology,
Hospital Eugenio Espejo, Quito Ecuador

INTRODUCTION

Parkinsonism has been defined as a complex syndrome with many etiologies. Parkinsonism is most common in the elderly, its cause is unknown and it is represented by idiopathic Parkinson's disease (PD) and other neurodegenerative conditions. PD is the most common cause of parkinsonism and accounts for about 75% of all cases [1]. Vascular parkinsonism (VP) is a type of a parkinsonism secondary to cerebrovascular disease. In population and clinical cohort studies, it accounts for 2.5-12% of all cases of parkinsonism [1-11]. When the diagnosis includes pathological and imaging studies, VP accounts for 3-6% of all cases of parkinsonism [12]. In a clinico-radiological study of patients with stroke who had deep cerebral infarctions and white matter lesions, it was observed that nearly a third of the patients had one or more parkinsonian signs one year after their stroke [13].

* Address: Dr Fernando Alarcón, Chief of Neurology Department, Professor of Neurology, Hospital Eugenio Espejo, Av Colombia s n, Quito Ecuador, E-mail: falarcn2000@hotmail.com, Phone:593 2 2221202

Edouard Brissaud suggested that Parkinson's disease was due to a lesion in the substantia nigra [2]. In 1929, Critchley made the first description of a type of parkinsonism in elderly patients with high blood pressure caused by cerebrovascular disease, which he called atherosclerotic parkinsonism [3]. He described the course of the disease in these patients as rapid and as preferably affecting the lower limbs, suggesting that multiple vascular lesions in the basal ganglia were presumably responsible for producing the cardinal symptoms in this syndrome. He classified it into five subtypes: 1) parkinsonian symptoms and short-stepping gait; 2) parkinsonism associated with pseudobulbar palsy; 3) parkinsonism with dementia; 4) parkinsonism with pyramidal tract signs; and 5) parkinsonism with cerebellar ataxia. The concept was accepted for decades, until it became controversial, because of the imprecision of its limits, the lack of pathological evidence and because it included heterogeneous conditions. Schwalb and England rejected the concept, [4] arguing that the evidence of vascular change found in some patients with PD could be an incidental finding. Afterwards, Critchley revised his initial concept and introduced the term “vascular pseudo-parkinsonism” to provide it with a broader meaning to vascular participation and to differentiate it from idiopathic PD [3-5].

The concept of VP continues to be discussed because of the absence of diagnostic criteria and because of the difficulty that there is, in some cases, in differentiating VP from PD [5, 6]. In addition, the patients included in the initial studies do not meet current criteria for Parkinson's disease. As a rule, however, there is an agreement to replace the term atherosclerotic by vascular because it would thus include ischemic or hemorrhagic lesions not caused by atherosclerosis [6].

The clinical presentation and background of cardiovascular disease (CVD) may be imprecise. Vascular lesions are frequently found in pathologically confirmed PD [7]. The diagnosis of VP is especially complex if we consider that, in elderly patients without parkinsonism, infarcts are frequently found in subcortical cerebral white matter and basal ganglia [5, 7, 8].

In patients with VP, brain imaging studies are useful for two purposes: to exclude other causes of degenerative parkinsonism (progressive supranuclear palsy) and to discard secondary causes (tumors, hydrocephalus) [14]. Computerized tomography (CT) and magnetic resonance imaging (MRI) have contributed to the concept of VP over the past few decades [15-22]. The presence of cerebrovascular lesions in basal ganglia or subcortical white matter in patients with parkinsonism suggests VP, although this does not exclude a diagnosis of PD [15].

Because of its broad spectrum, the clinical diagnosis of VP is complex. The definitive diagnosis of VP is neuropathological [23], although this is not specific because the changes found are those characteristic of small vessel disease and that is why there are doubts about whether VP should be identified as a clinical entity or as a clinical expression of small vessel disease or of an acute focal ischemic lesion [23, 24].

EPIDEMIOLOGY

In population studies, supported with clinical, imaging, and neuropathological findings, it has been found that between 2.5% and 12% of the cases of parkinsonism might have had a vascular cause [10, 11, 14, 27]. In a prospective population study conducted in Spain, which included 5,160 elderly subjects, VP accounted for 4.4% of all cases of parkinsonism identified during the period targeted by the study [8, 9]. A similar study conducted in Italy established a diagnosis of VP in 12% of patients [10]. The incidence of parkinsonism and PD has been found to be higher in elderly patients and men [7-11, 27]. In the Rotterdam study of a prospective population cohort, out of a total of 132 patients with parkinsonism, 5% had parkinsonism stemming from cerebrovascular disease [25]. In the survey of five European communities (EUROPARKINSON), VP was found in 3% of total cases of parkinsonism [26]. In epidemiological studies conducted in patients with PD, the prevalence of high blood pressure, heart disease and CVD is similar to, or lower than, that found in the control patients [18]. These results suggest that PD does not have a vascular origin. Therapy with levodopa could increase the levels of homocysteine, producing an impairment of the vascular endothelium and atherosclerosis, increasing the risk of ischemic cerebral events [20- 23]. Due to the absence of well-defined criteria and the wide clinical spectrum, the results of epidemiological studies on vascular parkinsonism are highly variable.

Autopsy studies of 100 patients diagnosed and treated for PD reported by Parkinson's UK Brain Bank confirmed Parkinson's disease in 76 cases. In 24 cases, however, pathological findings different from PD were found, including vascular lacunar state in 3 cases [7]. The post-mortem evidence showed one lacunar state without the pathological characteristics of PD [7]. In this series, in 19 patients with PD, it coexisted with striatal vascular pathology [7]. This autopsy report showed the clinical difficulty of differentiating patients with PD from those with other types of parkinsonism. The validity of the concept of parkinsonism secondary to CVD has been challenged, and this has made it all the more difficult to conduct epidemiological studies [24-28]. Despite these results, the general perception is that VP is being underdiagnosed [2-7, 12-24]. In our series of patients with VP examined in outpatient services, we found VP in 12% of cases [29]. In stroke patients admitted to the Neurology Department of the Eugenio Espejo Hospital, the frequency of parkinsonism amounted to 3% [30].

Clinical Characteristics

Cerebrovascular disease and parkinsonism secondary to drug use are the most important causes of secondary parkinsonism [1-27, 31, 32]. Vascular parkinsonism is a form of secondary parkinsonism stemming from an ischemic cerebrovascular disease and, exceptionally, hemorrhagic CVD. The concept of vascular parkinsonism is controversial and has been challenged, although recent studies have reinstated the concept as a clinical entity [24, 27, 31, 32]. PD and VP are common among the elderly and they often appear concomitantly [1, 16, 27]. Vascular parkinsonism has been described by many authors [2-4, 9, 13, 24, 27, 30-32] as a heterogeneous clinical entity that is difficult to define [32] and which may present symptoms similar to neurodegenerative diseases such as PD, supranuclear palsy, corticobasal degeneration, and other neurodegenerative disorders where tremor, rigidity, bradykinesia, and other parkinsonian signs are present [1, 6]. In some series, it was not possible to differentiate the clinical characteristics between VP and PD [31, 32]; nevertheless, some experienced neurologists have reported that it is indeed possible [33, 34]. PD can frequently be associated with cerebrovascular lesions [35, 36]. It is necessary to establish the signs and symptoms that have greater specificity for the diagnosis of VP because of their therapeutic and prognostic implications. Some series show that 20-25% of patients with PD show signs of cerebrovascular disease [23, 28]. In a study of 617 cases with a pathological diagnosis of PD, 56% of them did not show any cerebrovascular pathology, except mild to moderate amyloid angiopathy [28].

Clinical, pathological, and imaging findings suggest that VP and PD are different clinical entities [7, 24, 31, 36-40]. Several clinical criteria have been proposed to differentiate VP from PD [3-9, 12, 14, 26, 41-69]. Clinically, VP presents as an atypical parkinsonian disorder. In our series, we have recognized three types of vascular parkinsonism.

The first type of vascular parkinsonism is acute post-stroke parkinsonism (APSP), which accounts for 3.5% of patients with parkinsonism, and it is associated with infarcts in striate bodies and lenticular nucleus and, less frequently, with frontal or parietal, midbrain or cerebellar lesions [2, 4, 5, 13, 27, 29-32, 41-69]. APSP may be present in a unilateral or bilateral form with unilateral predominance. The age of onset is much later than in PD. In our series, the average age at onset of symptoms is 65 years old. The most important risk factor is high blood pressure. Hemiparkinsonism and ipsilateral hemiparesis usually occur concomitantly or after a stroke [24, 30, 31, 41, 49-53]. The infarction may be atherothrombotic, lacunar, cardioembolic or related with other etiologies. Exceptionally, patients may present hemorrhage [30, 31, 41, 51]. The type of vascular lesions may be heterogeneous, because of the occlusion of large, medium-sized or small intracerebral vessels.

The distribution of hypertonus in these patients suggests a lesion of the upper motor neuron affecting the anti-gravity muscles rather than the extrapyramidal pattern found in PD. Bradykinesia of a variable degree is often found with evidence of micrography in some patients [27]. Patients tend to present the affected side in a rigid-spastic form, which in some cases is accompanied by flexion and internal rotation of the forearm and hand, with a hemiparetic gait. Tremor at rest may be slow and accompanied by posture tremor. It tends to be monotonous such as in PD and may be more evident with arms outstretched [31, 52, 53]. Hemihypokinesia may be partially attributed to a pyramidal impairment; nevertheless, slowness of shoulder and amplitude reduction of the arm movement during walking are clearly more prominent than what could be expected from a pyramidal impairment [45]. The later onset of parkinsonian symptoms in patients with severe weakness because of an infarct of the anterior cerebral artery and observation that parkinsonism appears in the arm and not in the leg that is more affected suggest that extrapyramidal symptoms appear during recovery of the pyramidal impairment [45]. Hemiparkinsonism has been associated with damage to the supplementary motor area, the angular gyrus or frontal-subcortical areas that alter the interconnection of the tracts connecting the basal ganglia, thalamus, and motor cortex [30, 41, 52-61].

It has been proposed that, among patients with an infarct of the anterior cerebral artery, there would be a functional disconnection of the striate circuit-supplementary motor area [41]. Patients with APSP associated with infarcts that compromise the supplementary motor area may present improved motor function after severe weakness of the limbs [41]. It has been suggested that hemiparkinsonian symptoms secondary to a lesion of the brainstem would occur not only as a consequence of a defect of the nigral control over the ascending thalamocortical system but also as a result of the compromise of the descending reticular pathways that go to the motor centers of the brainstem and that would have their greatest impact in akynesia [36, 60]. Unilateral parkinsonian symptoms would be the result of an impairment in the connectivity between the thalamus and prefrontal area and the descendent projections to the basal ganglia [60, 63]. When it is bilateral, resting and posture tremor and ataxia, which may have a unilateral predominance, apraxia, episodes of motor blockage, short-stepping, and postural as well as gait instability may appear. It has been proposed that the pathogeny of unilateral or bilateral post-stroke parkinsonism would occur as a result of the impairment of the interconnection between the basal ganglia, the thalamus, and the motor cortex, which would lead to an impairment of sensory-motor integration and the descendent reticular pathways to the brainstem [31, 69].

APSP may be secondary to unilateral or bilateral infarcts of the basal ganglia, thalamus, midbrain, supplementary motor area, angular gyrus or frontal-subcortical areas, and cerebellum [2, 24, 29, 30, 40, 69-75]. Pathological changes in the cerebellum have been associated with PD [77]. In anatomical studies, reciprocal interconnections have been identified between the basal ganglia and the cerebellum [76]. Functional or morphological modulation of the cerebellum has been detected with respect to akynesia, rigidity, tremor, gait disorder, dyskinesia and some non-motor symptoms [77]. Tremor found in 75% of PD patients, when it is the generally predominant symptom, presents when the disease has a more benign course [78]. In pathophysiological terms, tremor is linked to abnormal activity of two circuits: the basal ganglia, which are primarily affected by the depletion of dopamine in PD, and the cerebellar-thalamocortical circuit, which is also compromised in other types of tremor [77, 78]. Resting tremor at the onset of the movement is not inhibited enough when the cerebellum is absent or not functioning well, suggesting that the cortico-cerebellar activation during voluntary movement suppresses the rhythm of the tremor [78]. The re-emerging tremor can be explained by the reinitiation of the cerebellar-thalamocortical tremor circuit through the basal ganglia [78]. Probably the larger role played by the cerebellum in PD includes pathological and compensatory effects [77, 78]. The pathological changes in the cerebellum can be induced from the basal ganglia by abnormal neuronal units or by dopaminergic treatment, which could be the cause of some clinical symptoms in PD [77]. The compensatory effect of the cerebellum can help to better uphold the motor and non-motor function in PD [77]. This could explain the absence or slight predominance of resting tremor in some cases of VP, where the circuit of the basal ganglia is often compromised, but cerebellar lesions are not often found. In our series, in few cases of APSP with cerebellar vascular lesions, the tremor was postural and kinetic. The response to dopaminergic therapy is good in most cases of APSP, especially when the patient has lesions in the striate bodies or in the areas close to the white matter that compromises the nigrostriatal pathway [24, 30, 31, 70]. In these patients, the picture of parkinsonism can appear early or late up to 12 months after the stroke [24, 29, 30, 31].

The second type of VP, which accounts for 6.9% of patients with parkinsonism, is the most insidious and with a gradually progressive course, associated in the MRI with hyperintense lesions and small lacunar infarcts of the subcortical white matter and other deep structures, including the striate bodies and brainstem [24, 29, 31]. This type of VP has been recognized as progressive vascular parkinsonism (PVP) [29, 69].

PVP is associated with vascular lesions of the subcortical white matter and other deep structures. The patients are elderly at the start of the extrapyramidal signs. In our series, the average age at the onset of symptoms is 72. The most important risk factor is high blood pressure. The symptoms of these patients are insidious, with atypical signs, gradually progressive course, and a tendency to be bilateral. Patients can present postural tremor and, exceptionally, tremor at rest, which on occasion is arhythmical. The gait is short-stepping, alteration of the lower limbs predominates, and there is early postural instability. Motor impairment is often progressive, with a tendency to present a festinating gait and early, frequent motor blockages as a prominent manifestation. The patients can present early or late delirium, hallucinations, pseudobulbar palsy, bilateral pyramidal signs, dysarthria, dysphonia, urinary incontinence, cerebellar signs, and cognitive impairment [24, 29, 30, 31, 67, 69]. Impairment of motor and cognitive functions in most cases can be severe as early as 10 years before the onset of the disease. Life expectancy is much shorter than for APSP and PD. In the MRI, extensive lesions of the subcortical white matter appear [24, 29, 30, 31, 67, 69], to which brainstem hyperintensities are gradually and progressively added, in most cases.. The patients often present early motor complications during dopaminergic treatment [2-6, 7-9, 12-15, 24, 36, 69, 70] which are different from and of less severity than in PD. Dyskinesias are early, predominating in the upper limbs, much less intense and disabling than in PD, and are located preferably in the hands and exceptionally at the axial level. Fluctuations are more erratic and less intense at the onset of the disease with a tendency to worsen rapidly [24, 69, 70]. In patients with PVP, the therapeutic response to dopaminergic treatment is erratic, with a tendency to worsen rapidly. After the second year, the response to treatment is poor and, after more than seven to eight years of the disease, most patients do not respond to treatment and therefore in more than one patient the dopaminergic medication is withdrawn [14, 69]. Before establishing that a patient with PVP does not respond to levodopa, a dosage of at least 1,000 mg per day for a period of no less than three months must be reached. The response to dopaminergic therapy is moderate in the first years, very poor in intermediate stages, and unnecessary in many cases in advanced stages [1, 14, 69, 70].

The third type of vascular parkinsonism, that is, recurrent post-stroke parkinsonism (RAPSP), which accounts in our series for 1.4% of patients with parkinsonism, appears when patients with APSP present recurrent strokes and, gradually and progressively, show bilateral symptoms accompanied by hemiparesis or tetraparesis, with pyramidal and extrapyramidal alteration and severe postural instability similar to that patients present with CDPP. The average age of patients with RAPSP is …. The highest risk factor is high blood pressure. Symptoms worsen rapidly with every new stroke. To the tremor that initially could have been resting tremor, is progressively added posture tremor and, in some cases, kinetic tremor. Progressively the predominant alteration occurs in the lower limbs with postural instability, requiring early assistance for some daily routine activities. Patients can present pseudobulbar palsy, bilateral pyramidal signs, aphasia, dysarthria, dysphagia, urinary incontinence, and cognitive impairment. Patients are in wheelchairs 7 to 9 years after onset of parkinsonism and die between 10 and 12 years after their first stroke. Response to the dopaminergic therapy although is at first good, it rapidly and gradually loses its effectiveness. Motor complications are less intense and disabling than in PD. The response to dopaminergic therapy is poor as the disease progresses, and this therapy is often unnecessary.

Several clinical criteria have been proposed to differentiate VP from PD [24, 31, 67, 76]. It is necessary to differentiate the different types of VP from PD. APSP is associated with an acute cerebral infarction, involving an average age that is older than for PD but younger than for PVP, and cerebrovascular risk factors are more prevalent than in PD. Usually its presentation is unilateral or bilateral with unilateral predominance; tremor is not frequent and can be resting or posture tremor, and there is hemiparesis with prominent hypokinesia of the shoulder and swinging and presents with an atypical parkinsonian disorder [14], occasionally with oral and hand dyskinesias, with upper motor neuron signs [14, 24, 29, 30, 31]. Exceptionally, they can recover spontaneously. When it is unilateral, it has characteristics that are very close to those of PD: When it is secondary to striatal infarcts, it has a clinical presentation that is very similar to PD. Patients with APSP have a tendency, in some cases, to stay unilateral for a longer time than in PD.

In patients with PVP, the clinical presentation starts gradually and its progression is insidious. It appears at a later age than for patients with APSP and PD. Patients very frequently have cerebrovascular risk factors, and predominant motor symptoms are in the lower limbs with a tendency to be bilateral. Posture is more erect than in PD, with a marked tendency to retropulsion, steps are usually short, tending to stick the tips of the feet outward and in some cases there is a mild cerebellar ataxia [3, 9, 12, 14, 24, 29, 31, 67]. Instability, motor blockage, and falls are important from the early stages of the disease [5, 6, 14, 31, 67]. Symptoms of the upper limbs are less prominent, the average of the motor segment of the UPDRS being greater in the lower limbs compared with the upper limbs [14]. Resting tremor has been reported in 13% of cases and postural tremor in a higher percentage of cases [8, 14]. In our series, the percentage of patients who had resting and posture tremor was higher than reported. Tremor at rest, when present, is different from that which is present in PD, and it compromises the hand more than the fingers, with a tendency to be broader and with a variable frequency. Muscle tone is normal when there is slow joint movement and increases with rapid joint movement. Lead pipe rigidity is predominant compared to cogwheel rigidity [14]. There may be signs of upper motor neuron, with spasticity, extension of the plantar reflex, and hemiparesis. Dysphagia, dysarthria, and emotional incontinence with senseless laughter or sobbing may be, in some cases, prominent signs of this type VP [14, 31, 67]. Dementia and downward gaze paralysis may be present, even though they are not frequent in the early stages. In addition, there may be cerebellar signs [8]. In our series, we have found some patients with stuttering, oromandibular and hand dyskinesias which appear early but are not associated with the dopaminergic treatment or the use of drugs. In most patients with VP, both APSP and PVP are progressive, although PVP is more severe and disabling. The patients with PVP need, in most cases, to lean on a cane after the third year of the disease, must walk with the support of a walker after the sixth or seventh year, and usually need a wheelchair after the eighth or ninth year, thus constituting the cane-walker-wheelchair syndrome that is characteristic of this disease. When patients need the help of a walker, their cognitive functions usually begin to gradually and progressively decline, which isall the more evident when the patient stays in a wheelchair.

The third type of vascular parkinsonism, RAPSP, appears in 27% of patients who had APSP and subsequently present new ischemic infarcts in basal ganglia or in the brainstem, cortex, subcortex or cerebellum. These patients evolved progressively towards a clinical presentation of PVP.

Furthermore, patients with PVP can present, in their evolution, acute cortical or subcortical infarcts in basal ganglia or in the brainstem that speed up motor and cognitive impairment. A partial or total recovery of certain patients with APSP or PVP could be related to brain plasticity and/or reinnervation [30].

In PD, the clinical symptoms are characteristically unilateral at the beginning and then progress to the opposite side. It is assumed that idiopathic PD accounts for between 60% and 75% of all cases of parkinsonism [1, 7, 34, 69]. The criteria established by the Parkinson's UK Brain Bank to diagnose Parkinson's disease include: bradykinesia and at least one of the following signs: muscle rigidity, tremor at rest between 4 and 6 Hz and postural instability not related to visual, vestibular, or cerebellar disorders or proprioceptive deficits [7, 33, 34, 37]. The predictive factors of a more rapid progression and a short survival time include older age at the onset of PD, associated comorbidities, presentation with rigidity and bradykinesia, and decline in the response to dopaminergic treatment [34]. They present tremor of the hand at rest as an initial manifestation in 75% of cases [1]. Steps tend to be short and parallel, while muscle tone increases when attention is distracted by provocative manoeuvres. The duration of PD is longer; the score on the UPDRS scale is lower than with VP, the response to levodopa is good; and the course of the disease is slowly progressive [24, 30, 64, 65, 70-72].

The presence of cerebral infarctions in asymptomatic elderly persons and in patients with PD confirmed pathologically contributes to increasing the difficulty in reaching a diagnosis of VP [7, 37, 73-75]. There are few post-mortem studies, as a result of which it is difficult to establish the incidence of cerebrovascular pathology in PD [7, 28, 37, 73, 77, 78]. A comparison has been made of 617 consecutive cases, in which Parkinson's disease was confirmed by autopsy, with 535 age-matched controls, where a total frequency of cerebrovascular lesions, lacunas, amyloid angiopathy, lesions in white matter, recent and old ischemic infarcts, and hemorrhages were found in 44% of patients who had PD and in 32.8% of the controls. However, hemorrhagic acute cardiovascular disease (ACVD) or, more often, fatal ischemic ACVD was found less frequently in patients with PD, compared to the controls, 1.8% compared to 2.6% [28]. In a series of 700 cases of parkinsonism, PD accounted for 80.7% of the cases. In this series, the coexistence of cerebrovascular lesions was found in 19% of the cases, mainly with changes in the subcortical white matter or lacunar infarcts in the basal ganglia, old infarcts in 14.2% and multi-infarct encephalopathy in 2.5% [28]. Patients with PD showed a higher percentage of mild and moderate changes, that is, 26.8% and 10.6% compared to 20.9% and 6.5%, respectively, whereas the severe changes were similar in PD and in the controls, 6.8% compared to 5.4%. Recent acute infarcts and cerebral hemorrhages were rare in PD and in the controls [28]. In another study of 200 autopsies of proven cases of PD, cognitive impairment was significantly related to the severity of the coexistence of the Alzheimer-type pathology [79]. Only a small group of patients with PD with severe cerebrovascular lesions showed a significant rise in cognitive impairment, regardless of the severity and extensiveness of the Alzheimer-type neuritic changes [79]. These results contradict those previously found in other studies [28, 35].

Criteria for PD are increasingly stricter and have contributed to improve its diagnosis [7, 33, 34, 37, 75, 80] which is basically clinical. It is important for therapeutic and prognostic reasons to differentiate PD from other forms of parkinsonism. Clinicopathological studies based on Parkinson's UK Brain Bank have shown that the clinical diagnosis of PD is correct in 76% of cases [7, 37]. In subsequent studies, it has been suggested that there has been an improvement in the diagnosis, from 84% to 90% [34, 37]. Most false negative cases corresponded to multiple system atrophy, but also to VP, among others [7, 34, 37]. Despite the rigorous application of the proposed clinical criteria, the false positive cases have remained at 10% of all cases. It is possible that movement disorder specialists may be sharper in diagnosing PD [37]. In addition to the clinical diagnostic criteria of PD [7], genetic studies and various auxiliary evidence such as PET and SPECT studies can help in reaching the diagnostic decision [81].

The criteria for a clinical diagnosis of VP include the concomitant presence of parkinsonism and cerebrovascular disease, as well as a linkage between the two disorders [24, 29, 30, 31, 69, 75]. The definitive diagnosis of vascular parkinsonism is established by the presence of parkinsonism with pathological findings of vascular lesions and the absence of Lewy bodies or depigmentation of the substantia nigra, although in a clinicopathological series, loss of nigral cells and substantia nigra was found [24]. It is necessary to exclude hydrocephalus and other degenerative diseases that could produce parkinsonism, as well as parkinsonism secondary to drug use and other causes [14, 27, 69]. Clinically, VP appears in most cases as an atypical parkinsonian disorder.

Vascular parkinsonism differs from PD because of the older age at which the extrapyramidal presentation occurs, the higher frequency of vascular risk factors, and for its abrupt or insidious onset, with a more rapid progression. In VP with white matter hyperintensities, it is more frequent to find bilateral alteration, bradykinesia of the lower limbs, postural instability, gait disorders, and early motor blocks. In PD, three out of four patients present, at the onset of the disease, resting tremor and unilateral parkinsonism [1, 2, 5, 6, 7, 8, 13, 24, 27, 29, 30, 31, 41, 81].

Imaging Studies

The term VP encompasses a heterogeneous set of clinical syndromes with parkinsonism as a predominant symptom, which in the imaging studies shows several types of ischemic cerebral lesions without any findings suggestive of other degenerative causes of parkinsonism [68]. For neurologists, differentiating VP from PD is a diagnostic challenge. The presence of vascular lesions that are apparently similar found in the brain imaging studies can be associated, in certain cases, with parkinsonism, although in other cases it cannot [14, 27]. The imaging studies can serve two purposes in patients with VP: firstly, to exclude other causes of parkinsonism, such as progressive supranuclear palsy, multiple system atrophy, and other secondary parkinsonism such as drug-induced parkinsonism, post-encephalitic parkinsonism, normal pressure hydrocephalus, space-occupying lesions, etc. [14, 68, 69, 82, 83]; and secondly, the image shows the ischemic lesions that substantiate the clinical diagnosis [14]. Lesions associated with vascular parkinsonism have been related to multiple lacunar infarcts in the basal ganglia and with small vessel disease in the subcortical white matter [6, 24, 29, 31, 69]. Nevertheless, there is no clarity in the literature to differentiate the three types of VP in the findings of the imaging studies, which is needed to recognize that multiple lacunar infarcts in the basal ganglia, brainstem or the cerebellum, as well as infarcts of the large arteries are related to post-stroke parkinsonism [30], since multiple lesions of the subcortical white matter are the most frequent finding in patients with PVP [21, 31, 69]. RAPSP is recognized for its ictal clinical recurrence and the finding of acute stroke in imaging studies.

Vascular lesions are clearly better shown in the MRI than in the CT. The MRI or CT image supports the VP diagnosis, although it is not conclusive [14]. Patients with VP show a higher number of infarcts when compared, in the diffusion/perfusion-weighted (DW/PW) MRI, with age-matched patients with PD [14]. It has been proposed that there is a correlation between the images found in the MRI and the type of parkinsonism. MRI studies use the intensity and frequency of lacunar infarcts and/or subcortical white matter hyperintensities (SWMH) as a medium to establish the differential diagnosis between VP and PD. Nevertheless, these MRI findings are controversial because of the absence of any pathological confirmation to establish a predictive value for them [5]. In our series, patients were initially diagnosed as APSP, and in the follow-up they presented new acute vascular events and the clinical presentation of parkinsonism was modified, becoming bilateral with characteristics closer to PVP than to APSP as initially viewed. The new vascular events showed up on the DW/PW-MRI, in addition to the initial infarcts, new cortical vascular lesions in the subcortical white matter, basal ganglia, brainstem or which compromised the large cerebral arteries. Furthermore, patients with PVP may present infarcts or cerebral hemorrhages in the years after the initial diagnosis. The presence of vascular disease in the imaging studies substantiates the diagnosis of VP, but does not establish a cause-effect relationship [27].

Imaging studies have compared the changes in the cerebral CT and/or MRI [6, 9, 11, 82]. MRI is more sensitive than CT in diagnosing ischemic cerebrovascular disease. Patients with VP are more likely to have an abnormal image, varying between 90% and 100%, compared with PD, which fluctuates from 12% to 44% [32]. The principal abnormalities include infarcts in multiple territories, lesions in the subcortical white matter and periventricular lesions in 75% to 90% in VP and in 7% to 16% in PD, and ischemic lesions in basal ganglia in 38% to 44% in VP compared to 4.6% to 8% in PD [6, 8, 9, 78]. Of patients with PD, 70% have normal MRI [32]. In a comparative MRI study, patients suspected of having VP had significantly more subcortical lesions than those with PD or high blood pressure (32). There are clashing reports about the frequency of association of vascular lesions isolated from the substantia nigra and VP [27]. In a study of patients with lacunar infarcts of the basal ganglia, a low percentage of parkinsonism has been found [2] and, in another study, in 38% of patients [45]. A correlation between the images found in the MRI, the clinical presentation and the type of parkinsonism has been proposed [13, 36]. From the imaging standpoint, two types of vascular parkinsonism are recognized: the first is the ictal type which pertains to APSP or RAPSP [5, 13, 29, 31, 65, 67, 69] and the second type pertains to vascular parkinsonism of insidious onset, which is related to hyperintense lesions of the subcortical white matter in areas bordering the vascular territories and other small lesions located in basal ganglia and brainstem [24, 30, 31, 67, 69]. In our series, we have found patients with APSP, who became patients with RAPSP and patients with PVP, which in the follow-up presented stroke with infarcts of the small penetrating vessels and, exceptionally, because of occlusion of the larger arterial vessels. In practice it is not always possible to distinguish whether the onset is ictal or insidious. The MRI findings show that the lesions that produce vascular parkinsonism can be located outside the basal ganglia [5, 29, 31, 69].

Functional imaging studies with positron emission tomography (PET), simple photo emission tomography (SPECT) and spectroscopy by MRI can help differentiate PD from VP [6, 61, 69, 84-96]. Studies with SPECT can be used as a support for the morphological image of the MRI/CT in diagnosing various parkinsonian syndromes [27, 87]. SPECT, using the dopamine transporter (DAT) in the functional imaging techniques, can help differentiate presymptomatic PD from VP [97]. The technique defines the integrity of the dopaminergic system and has its main clinical application in patients with mild, incomplete, or uncertain parkinsonism [97]. The DAT image is abnormal in PD, multiple system atrophy and progressive supranuclear palsy, The imaging studies with specific ligands for DAT provide a marker for presynaptic neural degeneration. Using this technique, the reduction of the degree of striatal connectivity has been correlated with the severity of the PD, but not in patients with VP [27, 98]. The study with the SPECT is one of the of the most widely used to differentiate degenerative parkinsonism from other parkinsonian syndromes where the symptoms or clinical course of the disease are unusual [99]. The cocaine derivative ^{123}I-FP-CIT binds the dopamine transporter (DAT) and acts on the striate as a good marker to differentiate presynaptic disorder from other types of parkinsonism [99]. The image with specific SPECT ligands for DAT (FP-CIT, beta-CIT, IPT, TRODAT) test a marker for presynaptic neural degeneration [45, 89]. On the basis of this technique, it has been demonstrated that the degree of striatal reduction was correlated with the severity of the disease in PD, but not in patients with VP [27]. Studies with SPECT using the β-CIT dopamine transporter have found greater reduction in the averages of fixation in the putamen and caudate in PD than in VP. This reduction is related to the severity of PD [6, 87, 88]. Furthermore, the left-right asymmetry of the striatal β-CIT transporter is more frequent in PD than in the controls or VP [5, 6, 89]. These findings suggest that the typical pattern of the presynaptic dopaminergic deficit found in PD is not present in most patients with VP [5, 68]; therefore this study with SPECT could help to differentiate VP from PD [68, 72]. Nevertheless, a recent study shows a reduction in the fixation of the β -CIT dopamine transporter in two patients with VP, similar to that found in PD, although the confirming pathological finding was not available [6, 89]. The image of the dopamine transporter (DAT) may be abnormal in VP if there is a focal infarct in the basal ganglia [6]. Ligands of the striatal dopamine D2 receptors have also been studied in VP and they have not been found to be significantly diminished [6]. In patients with Parkinson's disease binding of receptor D2 is not decreased, in contrast with patients with MSA who demonstrate a reduction in D2 receptors as occurs in PD [99]. Regional cerebral blood flow has been assessed with PET, using the steady-state technique with 150 patients with vascular dementia who developed parkinsonism. This study showed a decline in regional cerebral blood flow and regional metabolic averages for oxygen in the frontal and parietal cortex and in the striate [5]; more over, the oxygen average was increased in the contralateral striate on the most affected parkinsonian side. PET findings suggest that focal ischemic changes could contribute to the development of parkinsonism in patients with vascular dementia [5]. MRI studies use the density and frequency of the lacunae's or hyperintensities in T2 in white matter to achieve an average and reach a differential diagnosis between VP and PD; this, however, is controversial because of the absence of subsequent pathological confirmation [5]. In our series, % of patients with VP had subcortical white matter hyperintensities, whereas % of patients with PD showed these changes. We found hyperintensity in the brainstem, especially in the protuberance, in % of VP patients and % had changes in the basal ganglia and substantia nigra. MRI studies with spectroscopy in PV have shown a decline in the average NAA/CRE in the frontal cortex and putamen, which was not observed in PD [6, 91].

PHYSIOPATHOLOGY

Pathogenesis

The term cerebral vascular small vessel disease (SVD) refers to a group of pathological processes with various etiologies that affect the small arteries, arterioles, venules and capillaries of the brain. The consequences of small vessel disease for the cerebral parenchyma are, above all, the lesions located in the subcortical structure [100]. SVD is one of the most common causes of cerebrovascular disease. SVD related to high blood pressure is a common accompaniement of ageing, as well as amyloid angiopathy [100]. The characteristics found in neuroimaging include small subcortical infarcts, lacunae, white matter hyperintensities, perivascular spaces, microbleeding and cerebral atrophy. SVD may present as a stroke or cognitive decline or be asymptomatic. SVD may often coexist with neurodegenerative diseases and exacerbate cognitive impairment, physical disabilities, and other symptoms of neurodegeneration [101]. Progressive lesion of the brain's white matter may lead to a decline in the patient's quality of living [102]. The mechanisms that link small vessel disease with damage to the parenchyma are heterogeneous and not fully known. The hypothetical cascade of physiopathological events leading from the small vessel disease to brain damage may have ischemic and hemorrhagic consequences. The reason why certain blood vessel ruptures lead to greater hemorrhaging whereas others lead to microhemorrhages is unknown; it is believed that thickening of the vessel walls could be associated with microhemorrhages [100]. The pathogenesis and even the etiology of some ischemic lesions such as white matter lesions are more hypothetical. In ischemic lesions caused by small vessel disease, contraction of the lumen of the blood vessels is believed to lead to a state of chronic hypoperfusion of the white matter, which eventually leads to a degeneration of the myelinated fibers as a consequence of the repeated selective death of the oligodendrocytes. These ischemic mechanisms have been demonstrated in animal models [100]. Damage to the white matter is believed to be a form of incomplete infarct or selective necrosis similar to that described for neurons [100]. Alternatively, an acute occlusion of the small vessel is hypothesized as a putative mechanism for lacunar infarcts, which leads to focal and acute ischemia and complete necrosis of the tissues. This theory, put forth by Fisher, has yet to be proven [100]. Other mechanisms such as damage to the blood-brain barrier, focal subclinical inflammation, and apoptosis of the oligodendrocytes could be compromised in the so-called ischemic forms of small vessel disease and contribute to the final pathological profile [100].

Pathogenesis of VP is different depending on the type of parkinsonism. The vascular mechanism in post-stroke parkinsonism is different from insidious and progressive parkinsonism associated with chronic ischemic changes that preferably affect the subcortical white matter. A focal vascular lesion of the basal ganglia infrequently causes parkinsonism [103]. Parkinsonism can be exceptionally due to ischemic lesions of the substantia nigra [41, 42, 62, 64, 84, 96], and this has been confirmed pathologically in one single case [84]. Few cases of unilateral parkinsonism after an infarct in the territory of the lenticulostriate arteries have been reported [6, 61]. It has been suggested that large vascular lesions cannot explain the subtle contralateral changes in the striatopallidal direct and indirect pathways [61]. Contrary to the above, it has been proposed that, for a vascular lesion to produce parkinsonism, it must be large and compromise the medial and lateral lenticulostriate arteries, including the putamen and the external globus pallidus, respecting the internal pallidus, the motor cortex, and the motor pathway [6]. Nevertheless, in our series, we found patients with small focal striatal lesions that produce contralateral hemiparkinsonism. We have observed that the lesions in the basal ganglia tend to be larger in acute post-stroke parkinsonism than in cases of PVP [69].

The pathogenic mechanisms of lacunar infarcts are poorly understood [100, 101, 106]. The evidence substantiates the hypothesis that, in most lacunar infarcts, the vascular pathology is diffuse, even when the clinical and imaging manifestations are focal [93]. Lacunar infarcts can lead to artery-to-artery embolism, cardiogenic embolism, or stenosis of the large intracranial arteries with cortical compromise [93, 96, 104]. Lacunar infarcts due to emboli or stenosis of the middle cerebral artery are larger, possibly because the embolus or stenosis occludes the origin of the various lenticulostriate arteries at the same time. It has been suggested that parkinsonism associated with lesions of the subcortical white matter can be due to chronic and progressive ischemia [65, 67]. Nevertheless, spectrocopy studies with magnetic resonance imaging in patients with VP have not detected any metabolic signs of ischemia in the subcortical white matter or in the striate [90, 91], nor have they found any deterioration in cerebral circulation [105].

It has been proposed that there is a causal relationship between PVP and lesions in subcortical white matter. Probably multiple acute ischemic microinfarcts produce neural loss [15, 105]. It has been suggested that the neurons present a rapid alteration that triggers acute clinical symptoms, although the underlying ischemic process is gradual. These neural changes could manifest themselves as a change in electrical activity or as a drop of blood flow below 25 ml / 100 gr / min of brain tissue. The drop in blood flow may be gradual but the symptoms are sudden [93]. There is damage to the endothelium of the perforating vessels, a rise in the permeability of the blood-brain barrier, and the release of toxic substances to the perivascular tissue and the cerebral parenchyma [93]. How can this gradual process trigger a sudden lacunar infarct or how can it be explained that the symptoms of the lacunar infarct progress afterwards? It has been suggested that the composition of the interstitial fluid draining through the vascular endothelium of the perforating vessels reaches a critical level of abnormality where the axons stop transmitting nerve signals. Furthermore, it has been proposed that, because of a decline in flow in blood vessels with thickened walls, the exchange of nutrients and products of the metabolism is not adequate. This diffuse endothelial failure would contribute to the formation of lacunar infarcts and microhemorrhages that may be either symptomatic or asymptomatic [93, 106-108].

Subcortical white matter hyperintensities (SWMH) in the MRI are an imaging manifestation of small vessel disease. Autopsy studies have shown that SWMH correspond to a heterogeneous pathological substrate with variable degrees of demyelination, arteriosclerosis and glyosis [109-113]. At the end of the spectrum of small vessel disease, lacunar infarcts caused by a lesion of the thalamus-perforating, lenticulostriate, and paramedian pontine arterioles would be found [112, 114]. Incomplete lacunar infracts that are not cavitated and that may represent an intermediate stage between SWMH and totally cavitated lacunae have been described [111, 115]. These findings can be discriminated with the help of diffusion-weighted, using the apparent diffusion coefficient, capable of differentiating reversible ischemia from an infarct. Lacunar infarcts of the white matter often develop within a pre-existing SWMH. The lacunae of the subcortical white matter are small cavities that have been recognized as ischemic infarcts that can be produced by various pathogenic mechanisms [111, 112, 115-117]. Because the affected subcortical white matter belongs to a borderline territory and is therefore more vulnerable, it has been proposed that the vascular lesions develop slowly in an area with compromised blood perfusion [111, 114].

There is evidence that post-stroke parkinsonian symptoms are more frequent when the patient has previously had SWMH and high blood pressure [6, 30, 40, 118-120]. The lesions that can produce vascular parkinsonism may be located in any area of the cortical-subcortical-basal ganglia motor circuit [6]. The physiopathology of vascular parkinsonism fluctuates according to the type of lesion and the symptoms found. Development of an extrapyramidal profile would also depend on the degenerative changes that could develop in the substantia nigra after the infarct, as a result of an excessive excitatory influence produced by the loss of the GABA impulse inhibition [121]. This reinforces the hypothesis that suggests a complex dysfunction of the pathways of the basal ganglia [91]. Chronic ischemia would produce SWMH and the loss of striatal D1 receptors as a result of mechanisms of hypoxia or secondary excitotoxicity [6]. In post-mortem studies of patients with lacunar infarcts, a marked imbalance between the averages of the D1 beta-preprotaciquinine and D2 preproencephalin has been found in the striatal efferent pathway [96]. Chronic ischemia reduces the expression of the alpha-4 and beta-2 subunits of nicotinic acid receptors that would trigger the dopaminergic pathway [122]. In experimental studies, the transitory focal cerebral ischemia lasting one hour induces a marked depletion in parkin protein levels. This depletion precedes neuron death [101, 123]. In short, hypoxia-ischemia mechanisms may lead to a dysfunction of the pallidal-thalamocortical pathway, at both the presynaptic level (substantia nigra) and the post-synaptic level (striatal efferent pathway) [6].

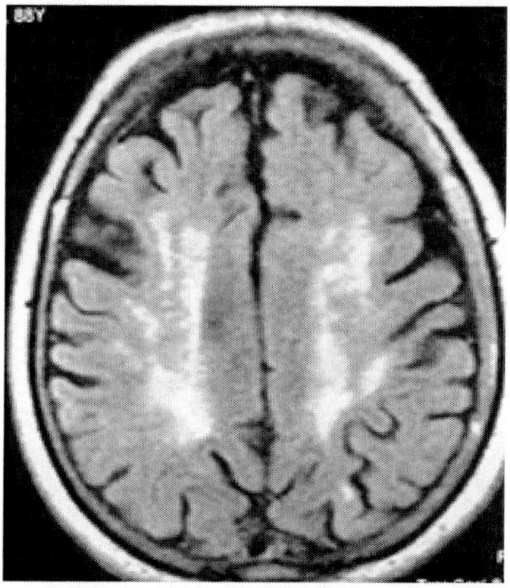

Figure 1. MRI, axial FLAIR view, shows hyperintense bilateral subcortical lesions.

It has been proposed that gait disorders appearing in VP patients are due to a deterioration in the executive and planning functions of the basal ganglia-frontal lobe circuit because of combined lesions of the subcortical white matter and the striate body (Figures 1A, 1B) [13, 102]. Nevertheless, recent clinical and experimental evidence indicates the participation of the pedunculopontine tegmental nucleus (PPN), which is a neurochemical and functionally heterogeneous structure holding a strategic position in the dorsal tegmentum of the midbrain and upper pons and contains cholinergic neurons, gamma-aminobutyric acid (GABA) and glutamatergic neurons, which receive direct impulses from the cerebral cortex and reciprocally with the basal ganglia and provide entries into areas of the motor thalamus, the brainstem and the spinal cord. These connections participate in controlling locomotion and muscle tone. PPN is affected in PD and atypical parkinsonian syndromes. The participation of PPN may play an important role in the impairment of gait in these disorders [124]. Recently, reduced connectivity of the PPN nucleus with the cerebellum, the thalamus and multiple regions of the frontal cortex has been reported; these structural and functional differences have only been found in the right hemisphere of parkinsonian patients with freezing of gait [125].

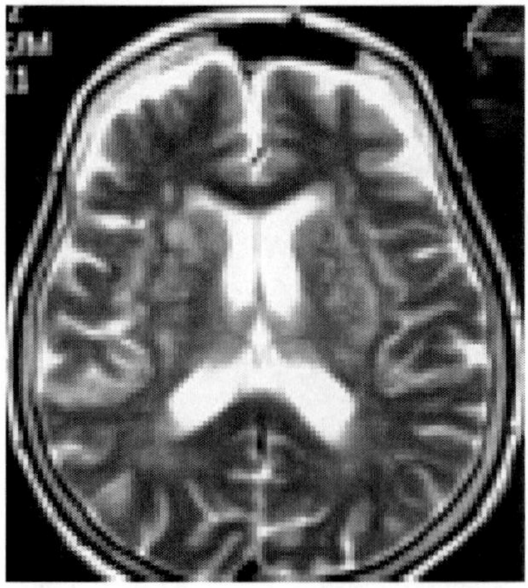

Figure 2. MRI, T2-weighted axial view, shows hyperintense ischemic lesions at the level of the basal ganglia at both sides.

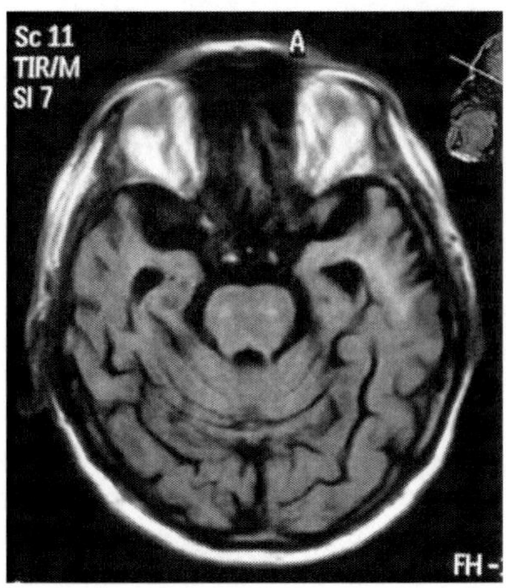

Figure 3. MRI, T2- axial FLAIR view, shows hyperintense lesions at the level of the pontine tegmentum.

Different challenges to the physiopathological concepts being proposed to explain VP have emerged: most patients with SWMH do not develop parkinsonism, and among patients with or without parkinsonism there is no difference in the severity of the vascular damage in basal ganglia and subcortical white matter. Some patients with infarcts or hemorrhages in the subthalamus, thalamus and ipsilateral cerebellum improved pre-existing parkinsonism [6, 126-128]. In the literature, cases of patients with hemiparesis-hemiballismus contralateral to the vascular lesion who subsequently developed parkinsonism ipsilateral to the lesion have been reported [119].

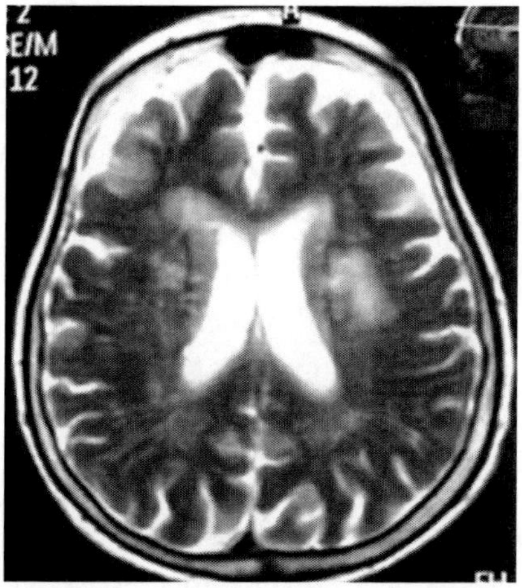

Figure 4. MRI, T2-weighted axial view, shows hyperintense bilateral subcortical ischemic lesions, most of which at the left semioval center.

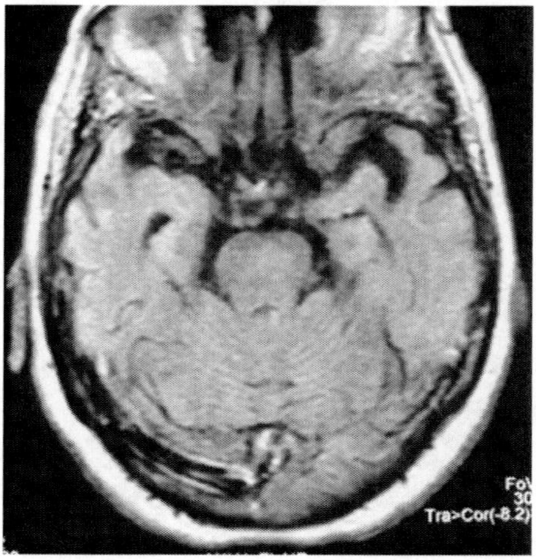

Figure 5. MRI, T1-weighted axial view, shows hyperintense hemorrhagic lesion, at the level of pontine tegmentum.

Small vessel disease is an important cause of age-related stroke, cognitive impairment, and disability. A better understanding of the pathogenesis of vascular injury and neural damage in the brain related to small vessel disease could help to better define the clinical consequences of these diseases and the frequency of the coexistence of different forms of small vessel disease such as lesions in the white matter, lacunar infarcts, and microbleeding [100]. White matter hyperintensities develop because of stenosis of multiple vessels, which can fluctuate from subtle ischemia to diffuse hypoxia or incomplete infarct. The lacunae's are caused by occlusion of the thalamus-perforating, lenticulostriate or paramedian pontine deep arterioles [129]. A subtype of lacunas that have not been cavitated and that can represent an intermediate stage between white matter hyperintense lesions and a totally cavitated lacunae has been described [129]. Subcortical lacunas that develop within pre-existing white matter lesions have been found frequently. It has been hypothesized that the lacunas of the subcortical white matter often develop slowly in the already compromised perfusion area [129]. As the subcortical white matter is an inflection action, it is more vulnerable to ischemia [100]. The direct origin of these arterioles from larger arteries can make them more prone to acute occlusion. Furthermore, the characteristics of the tissue may influence its survival, as the neurons of the deep gray matter can react to the ischemia differently from the glial cells of the subcortical white matter [100]. These findings suggest that the lesions of the subcortical white matter and the incident lacunas may have a pathogenesis that is different from the lacunas in the basal ganglia and the infratentorial region [100]. Therefore, patients with APSP, although they may have risk factors similar to those of patients with PVP, could be substantially different in their pathogenesis. Patients with PVP, because they are older than patients with APSP, could be more vulnerable to hypoxic ischemia in a gradual and progressive process that would compromise the glial cells of the subcortical white matter and would progressively affect the neurons of the basal and infratentorial ganglia. The follow-up studies with imaging in our patients with PVP show, gradually and progressively, small lesions in basal ganglia and diffuse lesions that progressively affect the brainstem, which would explain the bilateral alteration of lower limbs which is predominant and disabling in these patients. Exceptionally, we have found acute focal lesions in basal ganglia and brainstem in the context of this clinical profile.

The loss of integrity of white matter may be associated with gait disorders in small vessel cerebral disease [130]. Disorders of motor and cognitive control appearing in patients with PVP are probably a direct or remote effect of small vessel cerebral disease, which could interrupt the white matter tracts that interconnect bilateral cortical regions, especially the prefrontal cortex that is involved in cognitive control and motor performance [131]. In addition, blockage of gait, which causes frequent falls in patients with PVP, could be related to structural and functional deficits of the hemispheric motor network with a reduced structural connectivity between the pedunculopontine nucleus, the cerebellum, the thalamus and multiple regions of the frontal cortex [125]. Previous evidence shows why small vessel disease appears with various clinical manifestations, including VP, and why neurological impairment is different in patients with PVP.

In the clinical diagnosis of VP, three different clinical entities, which have parkinsonism and cerebrovascular disease in common, are recognized. The first is parkinsonism with at least one of the following signs: bradykinesia, tremor which can either at rest or postural, muscular rigidity or postural instability not caused by primary visual, vestibular, cerebellar or proprioceptive impairment. The second is cerebrovascular disease defined by evidence of relevant cerebrovascular disease from CT or MRI cerebral imaging studies or by the presence of focal signs or symptoms that are consistent with stroke.

Pathology

The criteria for the clinical diagnosis of VP are not widely accepted, because vascular lesions can coexist in patients with PD and VP or can be asymptomatic. The pathological confirmation of PD and VP is required [24, 76]. Pathological findings are deemed to be the gold standard for the diagnosis of VP, not only because they show vascular lesions but also because they can exclude PD and other atypical parkinsonisms such as synucleinopathies and tauopathies [14]. The most important pathological findings in VP are related to small vessel ischemic disease, lacunar infarcts, and occasionally infarcts of the larger cerebral arteries [14]. The clinical and neuroimaging data of patients suspected to have VP have been compared with those of patients who have PD, but the results are not conclusive [23, 32]. A diagnosis of VP may be difficult because many patients with Parkinson's disease concomitantly have cerebrovascular disease [28, 131]. The clinical-pathological correlation in patients with VP is different among patients with APSP, PVP and. RPSP. Patients with PVP are very closely related to lesions of the subcortical white matter, periventricular lesions, and lesions of the brainstem, whereas patients with PPS show lacunar infarcts in the basal ganglia, thalamus, cerebellum, frontal or parietal infarcts [27, 30, 69]. Patients with RAPSP start out as APSP and present subsequent ictal vascular events of the small, medium-sized or large arterial vessels. The macroscopic findings include variable degrees of cerebral atrophy, especially of the cortical sulci, and atherosclerosis of the large cerebral arteries [14]. The lacunar infarcts may be visible macroscopically or microscopically [14, 24]. Microscopically, loss of nigral cells can be found with severe damage in the lateral areas, with groups of slightly affected medial cells in the rostral portion of the substantia nigra [14, 24]. In a neuropathological study, extensive evidence was found of small vessel lesion in the putamen and globus pallidus [24], although in this study the type of vascular parkinsonism is not specified. Microscopically, the small vessel disease is associated with pathology which includes gliosis, perivascular paleness, arteriolar hyaline thickening, and rise in perivascular spaces [14, 24]. The coexistence between ischemic cerebrovascular disease and PD is well known [14] although the data are contradictory as some studies show a reduced risk of stroke over a lifetime and others indicate an increased risk of stroke [23]. The diagnosis, however, can be difficult and confirmation is only possible on the basis of a neuropathological examination, which still continues to be the gold standard to reach a final diagnosis of both Parkinson's disease and vascular parkinsonism [23]. The data support the concept that vascular parkinsonism is a clinical entity that is different, with distinct heterogeneous clinical and morphological characteristics.

Treatment

Because the term VP encompasses clinical syndromes that are not well defined and that include different pathogenic mechanisms, the therapeutic strategy may be different for each syndrome. In the two major recognized syndromes, when the patient has lacunar infarcts in the basal ganglia or in the medium or large arteries or when the patient has a diffuse small vessel disease, the response to levodopa may be different [29, 30, 69, 70]. The benefit of dopaminergic therapy tends to be higher in patients who have lesions in, or close to, the nigrostriatal pathway or in areas adjacent to the white matter. During the first months of treatment, the response does not show significant differences in the three types of VP. Nevertheless, during the following months and years, the response in the three types of VP is different. In most cases, patients with lacunar infarcts in the basal ganglia respond well to dopaminergic therapy and tend to respond like patients with PD, with a gradual and progressive loss of the therapeutic response to levodopa. The therapeutic response is upheld when there are no new cerebrovascular events. In these patients with APSP, the motor complications of dopaminergic therapy are less severe than in PD [36, 105], although in most cases they are present [36, 105]. Patients must be given physical therapy as a supplement to the pharmacological therapy. In patients with APSP, it is necessary to establish the etiology of the infarct and to control vascular risk factors such as high blood pressure, diabetes, cardiopathy, dyslipidemia, and others. For secondary prevention, in addition to controlling risk factors, antiplatelet and anticoagulant agents must be administered in cases of cardioembolism.

In patients with PVP, high blood pressure must be controlled as it is the principal risk factor, along with other risk factors for stroke. The response to levodopa tends to be initially good although in most cases there is a rapid deterioration in this response, as a result of which it is often necessary to increase the dose to at least one gram [5, 105]. In the advanced stage of patients with PVP and RAPSP when the response to dopaminergic therapy is very poor, the risk-benefit has to be assessed, especially when undesirable secondary effects are present, the dose may have to be reduced substantially and, in some cases, the dopaminergic therapy may have to be stopped altogether. In patients who show extensive lesions of the white matter in the MRI or multiple lacunar infarcts, it is reasonable to resort to antiplatelet agents [69]. It is often necessary to use acetylcholinesterase inhibitors for cognitive impairment. The use of atypical neuroleptics is indicated for episodes of confusion and hallucinations, and physical and cognitive therapy is recommended [69].

Most patients who, in their MRI, show extensive SWMH lesions with or without infarct respond poorly to levodopa. When these subcortical lesions are progressively associated with hyperintense lesions in the brainstem, the response to levodopa is even poorer and the degree of motor disability is even more severe, as these patients are marked by severe instability and freezing of gait. In MRI studies, it can be observed that lesions of the brainstem especially affect the protuberance and midbrain, compromising the dorsal tegmentum of the midbrain and upper pons where the pedunculopontine tegmental nucleus is located, which is one of the most important locomotor nuclei and has neurons related to the anticipatory postural adjustment preceding the initiation of stepping, as well as stepping itself, as a result of which it is critical for posture and coordination of walking to avoid freezing [124, 125]. In a recent publication, asymmetrical connectivity of the pedunculopontine network has been demonstrated in parkinsonian patients with blockage of gait. A strong association has been found between blockage of gait and frontal executive impairment. The hypothesis has been put forward that blockage of gait is associated with an interruption of connectivity between the region of the locomotor system of the midbrain and the frontal medial cortex; therefore, pedunculopontine lesions could be part of the dysfunction of the connectivity, regardless of the etiology of parkinsonism [125]. Affection of the peduncolopontine nucleus could play an important role in the deterioration of the gait of patients with PVP and RAPSP.

Because of the location of the lesions in APSP, the nigral neurons in most cases are preserved and the striatal cells and circuit of the basal ganglia are compromised, the basal ganglia start to deafferent from the thalamocortical pathways. This does not occur in Parkinson's disease, where the site of dopamine synthesis, the substantia nigra, is abnormal whereas the striate and the other parts of the basal ganglia are structurally intact. Patients with APSP who have infarcts in, or close to, the nigrostriatal pathways have a higher likelihood of responding to levodopa than those who have a disease of the white matter, because the dopamine administered exogenously can still be absorbed by the remaining neurons and can be converted into dopamine, which in turn can restore to a certain extent the dopaminergic connection between the cortical circuits and the structurally intact basal ganglia [14]. Patients with lesions in, or close to, the basal ganglia might show, in studies with SPECT, a poor taking of the ligands, and this can be a guide for treatment in APSP [14]. A positive response in patients with APSP can be explained by the presence of a remaining pool of striatal dopaminergic nerve endings in a dysfunctional nigrostriatal pathway that remains adequate to convert exogenous levodopa into dopamine and thus restore the intrinsic dopaminergic conduction. The absence of response to levodopa in other patients with nigrostriatal lesions may be because the increase in the exit of the basal ganglia as a result of the levodopa was unable to compensate for the dysfunction of the thalamocortical conduction [70].

Conclusion

Vascular parkinsonism continues to be a heterogeneous syndrome that is still not well defined. Patients with VP have more ischemic or hemorrhagic lesions, as well as SWMH and high blood pressure, than patients with PD. APSP, PVP and RAPSP must be differentiated, because of their therapeutic and prognostic implications. Mixed clinical presentations could be explained by the progressive profile and the broad physiopathological spectrum of cerebral vascular lesions.

In the criteria to establish a clinical and imaging diagnosis of VP, it is necessary to recognize three different clinical entities. Eventually, a fourth entity would have to be recognized, one that is associated with patients who initially present HSBS and subsequently present stroke events. All of these clinical conditions that constitute VP have parkinsonism and cerebrovascular disease in common. The first is parkinsonism with at least one of the following signs: bradiknesia, tremor which can be either resting or posture tremor, muscular rigidity or postural instability that is not caused by primary visual, vestibular, cerebellar or proprioceptive impairment. The second is cerebrovascular disease diagnosed by brain imaging studies in CT or MRI or by the presence of focal signs or symptoms that are consistent with stroke.

Among the criteria of exclusion, the following are noteworthy: history of repeated cranial trauma, encephalitis or other bacterial or parasitic infections, neuroleptic treatment or treatment with other medicines that may trigger parkinsonism at the onset of symptoms, presence of a brain tumor, communicating hydrocephalus or other alternative explanations for parkinsonism.

APSP is characterized by acute onset or delayed progressive onset where the imaging studies show acute lacunar infarcts and, exceptionally, hemorrhages in or close to areas that compromise the basal ganglia, the thalamus, the brainstem, the cerebellum and the frontal or parietal cortex. Parkinsonism in these cases may be similar to PD, starting up to a year after the stroke, at an age older than PD, as a unilateral or bilateral rigid-hypokinetic syndrome with frequent predominance ipsilateral to the motor deficit, the tremor may be resting, posture or, in a few cases, kinetic tremor. The response to levodopa and neurological impairment may progress similar to PD, as a result of which it is difficult, in many cases, to differentiate them if it is not possible to establish the ictal onset. The response to levodopa may be similar to PD, especially in patients with lesions in the basal ganglia and areas close to the white matter. Diagnosis is reached by the ictal onset and MRI findings of lacunas or small infarcts, especially in the basal ganglia and brainstem and, exceptionally, in large frontal, parietal or cerebellar vascular territories.

PVP appears in older patients, without any history of stroke, with high blood pressure as the most important risk factor. It is a clinical entity that begins insidiously with a slowing down in the initiation of voluntary movements with progressive reduction in speed and broadness of repetitive movements, which predominates in the lower limbs and progresses rapidly. It frequently comes with bilateral neurological signs and early cognitive impairment. In initial evaluations, patients show greater severity on the UPDRS scale compared to post-stroke parkinsonism and PD. At the beginning, in the MRI, they show subcortical white matter hyperintensities (SWMH) and, in some cases, lacunar infarcts. Afterwards the hyperintense lesions tend to be more extensive, with subcortical lacunar infarcts in the basal ganglia, brainstem, and less frequently in the cerebellum. This insidious and progressive presentation, in which vascular factors and chronic hypoxia with neural dysfunction and death intervene, severely and rapidly affecting the functional capacity of the patients, must be recognized as a different clinical condition.

RAPSP worsens the parkinsonian clinical condition of patients at each ictal episode with new ischemic lesions and, less frequently, hemorrhagic lesions. Parkinsonism in these patients is gradually progressive, tending to be bilateral and predominant in the lower limbs, accompanied by hemiparesis or tetraparesis, with pyramidal-extrapyramidal alteration and postural instability. The most important risk factor is high blood pressure. Symptoms worsen rapidly with each new stroke. Tremor may be resting, posture or kinetic tremor. The predominant alteration starts in the lower limbs with postural instability. They can present pseudobulbar palsy, bilateral pyramidal signs, aphasia, dysarthria, dysphagia, urinary incontinence and cognitive impairment. The MRI shows acute vascular infarct or hemorrhage at each ictal episode and, less frequently, hyperintense lesions in the subcortical white matter. Response to the dopaminergic therapy, which is initially good, is very poor as the disease advances and, in many cases, it becomes unnecessary. RAPSP refers to a percentage of patients who present repeated events of stroke, gradually and progressively evolving toward PVP. In addition, the pictures of PVP can be accompanied by ictal episodes with acute infarcts and hemorrhages. These "mixed" forms would be related to the broad atherosclerotic physiopathological spectrum and its clinical manifestations. We find these "mixed" pictures in very elderly patients, with a picture of Parkinsonism of the lower half of the body which predominates on the paretic side.

References

[1] Thomas M, Jankovic J. Clinical Diagnosis of Vascular Parkinsonism and Nondegenerative Atipical Parkinsonian Disorders En Atipical

Parkinsonian Disorders: Clinical and Research Aspects, Litvan I y Agid Y Eds, Totowa, New Jersey, Human Press Inc, 2005.

[2] Murrow RW, Schweiger G D, Kepes J J, Koller W C. Parkinsonism due to a basal ganglia lacunar state: Clinico pathologic correlation *Neurology* 1990;40:897-900.

[3] Crithely M. Arteriosclerotic parkinsonism *Brain* 1929;52:23-83.

[4] Eadie MJ, Sutherland JM. Aterosclerosis in Parkinsonian *J. Neurol. Neurosurg Psychiatry* 1964;27:237-24.

[5] SibonI, Tison F. Vascular parkinsonism. *Curr. Opin. Neurol.* 2004;17:49-54.

[6] SibonI, Fenelon G, Quinn NP TisonF.Vascular Parkinsonism. *J. Neurol.* 2004;251:513-524.

[7] Hughes A J, Daniel S E, Blankson S, Lees A J.A clinico pathologic study on 100 cases of Parkinson's disease. *Arch. Neurol.* 1993;50:140-148.

[8] Benito - Leon J, Bermejo - Pareja F, Rodríguez J, Molina JA, Gabriel R, Morales JM. Prevalence of PD and other types of parkinsonism in three elderly populations of central Spain. *Mov. Disord.* 2003;18:267-274.

[9] Benito - Leon J, Bermejo – Pareja F, Morales Gonzalez JM, Porta Etessan J, Trincado R, Vega S, Louis ED; for the Neurological Disorders in Central Spain (NEDICES)Study Group. Incidence of Parkinson‘s disease and parkinsonism in three elderly populations of central Spain. *Neurology* 2004;62:734-741.

[10] Baldereshi M, Carlo A, Rocca WA, et al. for the ILSA Working Group. Parkinson's disease and parkinsonism in a longitudinal study. Two fold higher incidence in men. *Neurology* 2000;55;1358-1363.

[11] Foltynie T, Barker R, Brayne C. Vascular Parkinsonism: a review of the precision and frecuency of the diagnosis *Neuroepedemiology* 2002;21:1-7.

[12] Bower JH, Dickson DW, Taylor L, Maraganore DM, Rocca WA. Clinical correlates of the pathology underlying parkinsonism: a population perspective. *Mov. Disord* 2002; 17:910-6.

[13] van Zagten M, Lodder J, Kessels F. Gait disorders and parkinsoniansgns in patients with stroke related to small deep infarcts and white matter lesions. *Mov. Disord* 1998;13:89-95.

[14] Gupta D, Kuruvilla A. Vascular Parkinsonism: what make it different? *Postgrad Med. J.* 2011; 87:829-836.

[15] Zijlmans J C M, Thijssen HOM, Vogels O J M, Kremer HPH, Poels PJE, Schooderwaldt H C, Merx LJ, HofMA, Thien T, Horstink MW.

MRI in patients with suspected vascular parkinsonism. *Neurology* 1995;45:2183-2188.

[16] Rosano C, Aizenstein HJ, Wu M et al. Focal atrophy and cerebrovascular disease increase dementia risk among cognitively normal older adults. *J. Neuroimaging* 2007;17:148-155.

[17] Appel J, Porter E, Bhatia N et al. Association of white matter hyperintensity measurements on brain MRI imaging with cognitive status, medial temporal atrophy and cardiovascular risk factors. *AJNR Am. J. Neuroradiol* 2009;30:1870-1876.

[18] Jerakathil T, Wolf PA, Beiser A, et al. Stroke risk profile predicts white matter hyperintensity volume: The framinghan study. *Stroke* 2004;35:1857-1861.

[19] Scherfler C, Scharz J, Antonini A et al. Role of DAT–SPECT in the diagnosis work up of parkinsonism. *Mov. Disor.* 2007;22:1229-1238.

[20] Kagi G, Bhatia KP, Tolosa E. The role of DAT-SPECT in movement disorders. *J. Neurol. Neurosurg Psychiatry* 2010;81:5-12.

[21] Zijlmans JC, The role of imaging in the diagnosis of vascular parkinsonism. *Neuroimaging Clin N Am* 2010;20:69-76.

[22] Zijlmans JC, Evans A, Fontes F, et al. (123) PF-CITSPECT study of vascular Parkinsonism and Parkinson's disease. *Mov. Disor.* 2007; 22:278-285.

[23] Jellinger KA. Vascular parkinsonism – neuropathological findings. *Acta Neurol. Scand.* 2002;105:414-415.

[24] Zijlmans J CM, Daniel SE, Hughes AJ, Revesz T, Lees A J. Clinico pathological investigation of vascular parkinsonism, including clinical criteria for diagnosis. *Mov. Disord.* 2004;19:630-640.

[25] De Lau LM, Giesbergen PC, de Rijk MC et al. *Incidence of parkinsonismo and Parkinson disease in a general population: the Rotterdam Study Neurology* 2004;63:1240-1244.

[26] De Rijk MC, Tzourio C, Breteler MM, el al. Prevalence of parkinsonismo and Parkinson's disease in Europe: the EUROPARKINSON Collaborative Study .European Community Concerted Action on the Epidemiology of Parkinson's disease. *J. Neurol. Neurosurg Psychiatry* 1997; 62: 10-15.

[27] Thanvi B, Lo N, Robinson T. Vascular parkinsonism –an important cause of parkinsonism in older people. *Age Ageing* 2005;34:114-119.

[28] Jellinger KA. Prevalence of cerebrovascular lesions in Parkinson's disease. A postmortem study. *Acta Neuropathol.* 2003;105:415-419.

[29] Alarcon F, Salinas R, Laguasi W, Maldonado JC, Dueñas G. Vascular parkinsonism: New classification proposal. *Movement Disorders*, 2009; Vol. 24, Suppl. 1:S 397 398.

[30] Alarcón F, Ziljmans JCM, Duenas G, Cevallos N. Post-stroke movement disorders: report of 56 cases. *J. Neurol. Neurosurg.* Psychiatry 2004;75:1568-1574.

[31] Winikates J, Jankovic J. Clinical Correlates of Vascular Parkinsonism. *Arch. Neurol.* 1999;56: 98-102.

[32] Demirjiran M, Bozdemir H, Sarica y. Vascular parkinsonism: a distinct, heterogeneous clinical entity *Acta Neurol. Scand.* 2001;104:63-67.

[33] Hughes AJ, Daniel SE, Kilford L, Lees AJ. The accuracy of diagnosis of parkinsonian syndromes in a specialist movement disorder service. *Brain* 2002; 125: 861 – 870.

[34] Hughes AJ, Ben – Shlomo Y, Daniel SE, Lees AJ. What features improve the accuracy of clinical diagnosis in Parkinson's disease: A clinicopathologic study. *Neurology* 1992; 42: 1142-1145.

[35] Mastaglia FL, Johnsen RD, Kakulas BA. Prevalence of stroke in Parkinson´s Disease A Postmorten Study. *Mov. Disord.* 2002 17 772 774.

[36] Jellinger KA. Overviewof morphological changes in Parkinson's disease *Adv. Neurol.* 1996;45:1-18.

[37] Hughes AJ, Daniel SE, Lees AJ. Improved accuracy of clinical diagnosis of Lewy body Parkinson's disease. *Neurology* 2001; 57:1497-1499.

[38] Calne BD, Snow BJ, Lee C. Criteria for diagnosing Parkinson's disease. *Ann. Neurol.* 1992;32: (Suppl)S125-S127.

[39] Gelb GJ, Oliver E, Gilman S, Diagnostic Criteria for Parkinson's disease. *Arch. Neurol.* 1999;56:33-39.

[40] Katzeschlager R, Zijlmans J, EvansA, Watt H, Lees AJ. Olfactory function distinguishes vascular parkinsonism from Parkinson's disease. *J. Neurol. Neurosurg Psychiatry* 2004;75:1749-1752.

[41] Kim JS. Involuntary Movement After Anterior Cerebral Artery Territory infarction. *Stroke* 2001;32:258-261.

[42] Akyol A Akyildiz U O, Tataroglu C. Vascular parkinsonism: A case of lacunar infarction localized to masencephalic substantia nigra. *Parkinsonism and Rel. Disord.* 2006;12:459-461.

[43] Morgan J C, Sethi KD. Midbrain infarct with parkinsonism. *Neurology* 2003;60:E10.

[44] Peralta C, Werner P, Holl B, Kiechl S, Willeit J, Sepi K, Wenning G, Poewe W. Parkinsonism following striatal infarcts incidence in a prospective stroke unit cohort. *J. Neural Trans* 2004;111:1473-1483.

[45] Reider - GroswasserI, Bornstein N M, Korczyn AD. Parkinsonism in patients with lacunar infarcts of the basal ganglia. *Eur. Neurol.* 1995;35:46-49.

[46] Piccini P, Pavese N, Canapicchi R, Paoli C, Del Dotto P, Puglioli M, Rossi G, Bonuccelli U. White matter hyperintensities in Parkinson's disease. *Arch. Neurol.* 1995; 52:191-194.

[47] Rampello M, Alvano A, Battaglia G, Raffaele R, VecchioI, Malaguarnera M. Different clinical and evolutional patterns in late idiopathic and vascular parkinsonism. *J. Neurol.* 2005; 252:1045-1049.

[48] Chang CM, Yu YL, Ng HK, et al. Vascular pseudoparkinsonism. *Acta Neurol. Scand.* 1992;86:588-592.

[49] Nagarattnam N, Davies D, Chen F. Clinical effects of anterior cerebral artery infarction. *J. Stroke Cerebrovasc. Dis. 1998*; 7: 391 – 397.

[50] Goldberg G, Mayer NH, Toglia JU. Medial frontal cortex infarction and the silent hand sign. *Arch. Neurol.* 1981; 38: 683-686.

[51] Balash Y, Korczyn AD Vascular parkinsonism. En Handbook of Clinical Neurology, Vol 84. Parkinson's disease and related disorders, Part II, W C Koller E Melamed Eds, Elsevier B V 2007.

[52] Dick JP, Benecke R, Rothwell JC, Day BL, Marsden CD. Simple and complex movements in a patient with infarction of the right supplementary motor area. *Mov. Disord* 1986;1:255-266.

[53] Jurgens U. The efferent and afferent conections of the supplementary motor area. *Brain Res.* 1984; 300: 63-81.

[54] Peters E, Eising EG, Przuntek Muller T. Vascular Parkinsonism: a case report and review of literature *Clin. Neurosci.* 2001;8:268-271.

[55] Inzelberg R, Bornstein NM, Reider I, Korczyn AD. Basal ganglia lacunes and parkinsonism. Neuroepidemiology 1994;13:108-112.

[56] Fujimoto K-i. Vascular Parkinsonism. *J. Neurol.* 2006;253 (Supl 3) III /16-III/ 21.

[57] Playford ED, Passingham RE, Nutt J, Frackowiac RSJ, Brooks DJ. Impaired activation of medial frontal areas during movement in Parkinson's disease: a PET study. *J. Cereb. Blood Flow Metab.* 1991;11(suppl):S1. Abstract.

[58] Kulisevsky J, Berthier MI, Avila A, Roig C. Unilateral Parkinsonism and stereotyped movements following a right Lenticular Infarction. *Mov. Disord.* 1996;11:752-754.

[59] Krauss JK, Grossman RG, Jacovic J. Improvement of Parkinsonism Signs After Vascular Lesions of the Basal Ganglia Circuitry. *Mov. Disord.* 1997;12:124-126.

[60] Kulisevsky J, Avila A, Berthier ML. Bipolar Affective Disorder and Unilateral Parkinsonism After a Brainsten Infarction. *Mov. Disord.* 1995;10:799-802.

[61] Fenelon G, Houeto J. Unilateral parkinsonism following a large infarction the territory of the lenticulostriate arteries. *Mov. Disord.* 1997;12:1086-1090.

[62] De la Fuente Fernandez R, Lopez J M, Rey del Corral P De la Iglesia Martinez. Peduncularhallucinosis and right hemiparkinsonism caused by left mesencephalic infarction. *J. Neurol. Neurosurg. Psychiatry* 1994;57:870.

[63] Defer G L, Remy P, Malapert D Ricolfi F, Samson Y, Degos J D.Rest tremor and extrapyramidal symptoms after midbrain haemorrhage: clinical and 18-F-dopa PET evaluation. *J. Neurol. Neurosurg. Psychiatry* 1994;57:987-989.

[64] Tolosa ES, Santamaria J. Parkinsonism and basal ganglio infarcts. *Neurology* 1984; 34: 1516-1518.

[65] Thompson PD, Marsden CD.Gait disorderof subcortical arteriosclerotic encephalopathyy Binswanger disease *Mov. Disord* 1987 2 1 8.

[66] Friedman A, Kang VJ, Tatemichi TK, Burke RE.A case of parkinsonism following striatal lacunar infarct ion. *J. Neurol. Neurosurg. Psychiatry* 1986 49 1087 1088.

[67] Fitzgerald PM, Jankovic J.Lower body parkinsonism evidence of vascular etiology. *Mov. Disord.* 1989 4 249 260.

[68] Benito Leon J, Bermejo Pareja F, Rodriguez J, Molina JA, Morales GR. Vascular Parkinsonism a clinical review. *Eur. Neurol.* 2009 61 11 15.

[69] Alarcon F. Parkinsonismo vascular. In Parkinson: Update and Review. M Rueda y L J Ruiz Eds. Asociasion. Colombiana de Neurologia. Editorial Kimpres, Bogota, 2009.

[70] Zijlmans JCM, Katzenchlager R, Daniel SE, Lees AJ. The L-dopa response in vascular Parkinsonism. *J. Neurol. Neurosurg. Psychiatry* 2004;75:545-547.

[71] Lee MS, Lee SA, Heo JH, Choi IS.A patient with a resting tremor and a lacunar infarction at the Border Between the thalamus and the Internal Capsule. *Mov. Disord.* 1993 8 244 246.

[72] Nagaratnam N, Kalasabail G. Contralateral abolition of essential tremor following a pontine stroke. *J. Neurol. Scienc.* 1997; 149: 195-196.

[73] Tan EK, Chan LL, Auchus AP. Complex Movement Disorders following bilateral paramedian thalamic and bilateral cerebellar infarcts. *Mov. Disord.* 2001 16 968 970.

[74] Kumral E, Evyapan D, Balkir K. Acute caudate vascular lesions, *Stroke.*! 999 30 100 108.

[75] Kalra S, Grosset DG, Benamer HTS. Differentiating Vascular Parkinsonism from Idiopathic Parkinson´s disease. A Systematic Review. *Mov. Disord. 2010* 25 149 156.

[76] Glass PG, Lees AJ, Bacellar A, Zijlmans J, Katzenschlager R, Silveira Moriyama L. The clinical features of pathologically confirmed vascular Parkinsonism. *J. Neurol. Neurosurg. Psychiatr*y 2012 83 1027 1029.

[77] Wu T, Hallet M. The cerebellum in Parkinson´s Disease. *Brain* 2013 136 696 709.

[78] Helmich RC, Hallet M, Deuschl G, Toni I, Bloem BR. Cerebral causes and consequences of parkinsonian resting tremor a tale of two circuits. *Brain* 2012 1 1 21.

[79] Jellimger KA, Attems J. Prevalence of cerebrovascular lesions in Alzheimer disease. A postmorten study. *Acta Neuropathol.* 2003 105 14 17.

[80] Suchowersky O, Reich S, Perlmutter J, Zesiewicz T, Gronseth G, Weiner WJ. Practice Parameter: Diagnosis and prognosis of new onset Parkinson disease (an evidence-based review) Report of the Quality Standards Subcommittee of the American Academy of Neurology. *Neurology* 2006; 66: 968-975.

[81] Tolosa E, Wenning G, Poewe W. The diagnosis of Parkinson's disease. *The Lancet Neurol.* 2006; 5: 75-86.

[82] Perez Saldana MI, Perez Velasco R, Burguera JA. Diagnostico del parkinsonismo vascular correlacion de la clínica con la neuroimagen y la utilidad de la SPECT con 123 I ioflupano.

[83] Alarcón F, Dueñas G, Lees AJ. Encephalitis Lethargica Due to Epstein Barr virus. *Mov. Disord.* 2011; 26: 2132-2134.

[84] Hunter P, Smith J, Thompson T, Dayan AD. Hemiparkinsonism with infarction of the ipsilateral sustancia nigra. *Neupathol. Apll Neurobiol.* 1978; 4: 297-301.

[85] Morgan JC, Sethi KD. Midbrain infarct with parkinsonism. *Neurology* 2003; 60: E10.

[86] Goldstein S, Friedman JH, Inis R, Seibyl J,Marck K .Hemi Parkinsonism Due to a Midbrain Arteriovenous Malformation Dopamine Transporter Imaging. *Mov. Disord.* 2001; 16: 350-353.

[87] Heiss WD, Wurker M. Value of functional imaging in Parkinson's disease and related movement disorders. *Nervenarzt* 1999 70 Suppl 1: s2- s10.

[88] BruckeT, Djamshidian S, Benesits .SPECT and PET imaging of the dopaminergic systemin Parkinson´s. disease. *J. Neurol.* 2000 247 Suppl 4 IV 2 7.

[89] Gerschlager W, Bencsits G, Pirker W, et al. [123I]beta-CIT SPECT distinguishes vascular parkinsonism from Parkinson's disease. *Mov. Disord* 2002; 17:518-23.

[90] Tzen KY, Lu CS, Yen TC, Wey SP, Ting G. Differential diagnosis of Parkinson´s disease and vascular parkinsonism by (99)TC-TRODAT. I. *J. Nucl. Med.* 2001;42:408-413.

[91] Zijlmans JC, de Koster A, van ¨Hef Ma, Thijssen HO, Hortsnk MW, Heerschap A. Proton magnetic resonance spectroscopyin suspected vascular ischemic parkinsonism. *Acta Neurol. Scand.* 1994;90:405-411.

[92] Abe K, Terakawa H, Takanashi M, et al. Proton magnetic resonance spectroscopy of patients with parkinsonism. *Brain Res. Bull* 2000; 52:589-95.

[93] Bhatia KP, Marsden CD. The behavioural and motor consequences of focal lesions of the basal ganglia in man. *Brain* 1994;117:859-876.

[94] Wardlaw JM. What causes lacunar stroke? *J. Neurol. Neurosurg. Psychiatry* 2005;76:617-619.

[95] Samuelsson M, Saderlfeld B, Olsson Gb. Functional outcome in patients with lacunar infarction *Stroke* 1996; 27:842-846.

[96] Schmidt R, Enzinger C, Ropele S, Schmidt H, Fazekas F. Progression of cerebral white matter lesions: 6-year results of the Austrian Stroke Prevention Study. *Lancet* 2003; 361:2046-8.

[97] Tohgi B, Utsugisawa K, Yoshimura M, Yamagata M, Nagane Y, Sayito K. Redustion in the ratio of beta-prepo tachykinintopro encephalin messenger RNA expression in postmortem human putamen during aging and in patients with status lacunaris. Implications for the susceptibility to parkinsonism. *Brain Res.* 1997;798:86-90.

[98] Marshall V, Grosset D. Role of dopamine transporter imaging in routine clinical practice, *Mov. Disord.* 2003; 18: 1415-1423.

[99] Gerschlager W, Bencsits G, Pirker W, et al. [123I]beta-CIT SPECT distinguishes vascular parkinsonism from Parkinson's disease. *Mov Disord* 2002; 17:518-23.

[100] Benitez-Rivero S, Marín-Oyaga VA, Garcia Solis D, Huertas Fernandez I, Garcia- Gomez FJ, Jesús S, Caceres MT, Carrillo F, Ortiz AM,

Carballo M, Mir P. Clinical features and 123 I FP SPECT imaging in vascular parkinsonism and Parkinson's disease. J. Neurol. *Neurosurg Psychiatry* 2013; 84: 122-129.

[101] Booth T.C., Nathan M., Waldman A.D., Quigley A.-M., et al. *The Role of Functional Dopamine-Transporter SPECT Imaging in Parkinsonian Syndromes,* Part 2. AJNR 2015, www.ajnr.org.

[102] Pantoni L. Cerebral small vessel disease: from pathogenesis and clinical characteristics to therapeutic challenges. *Lancet Neurol* 2010;9: 689-701.

[103] Wardlaw JM, Smith EE, Biessels G, Cordonnier Ch, et al. Neuroimaging standars for research into small vessel disease and its contribution to ageing and neurodegeneration . *Lancet Neurol* 2013;12:822-838.

[104] Potter GM, Marlborough FJ, Wardlaw JM. Wide variation in definition, detection, and description of lacunar lesions on imaging. *Stroke* 2010; 42: 359–66.

[105] Bhatia KP, Marsden CD .The behavioural and motor consequences of focal lesion of the basal ganglia nin man. *Brain* 1994;117:859-976.

[106] Voisin T. Raus de Feneryrols, Le Troon A. Cognitive impairment after first lacunar stroke: Clinical features and risk factors. *Cerebrovasc. Dis.* 2002;13(Suppl 3):297.

[107] Meguro K, Hatazawa J, Yamaguchi T, et al. Cerebral circulation and oxygen metabolism associated with subclinical periventricular hyperintensity as shown by magnetic resonance imaging. *Ann. Neurol.* 1990;28:378-383.

[108] Nakamura K, Saku Y, Ibayashi S, Fujishima M. Progrssive motor déficits in lacunar infarction. *Neurology* 1999;52:29-33.

[109] Kato H, Izumiyama M, Izumiyama K.silent cerebral microbleeds on T2 weighted MRI. Correlation with stroke subtype, stroke recurrence and leukoaraiosis. *Stroke* 2002;33:1536-1540.

[110] Wardlaw JM, Sandercock PA, Dennis MS, Starr J. Is breakdown of the blood-brain barrier responsible for lacunar stroke, leukoaraiosis and dementia? *Stroke* 2003;34:806-812.

[111] Pathological correlatesol late-onset dementia in a multicentre, community-based-population in England and Wales. Neuropathology Group of the Medical Research Council Cognitive Function and Ageing Study(MRC.CFAS) *Lancet* 2001;357:169-175.

[112] Fernando MS, Ince PG. Vascular Pathologies and cognition in a population –based cohort of elderly people. *J. Neurol. Sci.* 2004;226:13-17.

[113] AA,van der Flier WM, Fazekas F, et al. Progression of white matter hyperintensities and incidence of new lacunes over a 3-year period :The Leukoaraiosis and Disability Study. *Stroke* 2008;39:1414-1420.

[114] Jellinger KA. The enigma of vascular cognitive disorder and vascular dementia. *Acta Neuropathol.* (Berl) 2007;113:349-388.

[115] Roman GC, ErkinjuntiT, Wallin A, Pantoni I, Chui HC. Subcortical ischemic vascular dementia. *Lancet Neurol.* 2002;1:426-436.

[116] Chui HC. Subcortical ischemic vascular dementia. *Neurol. Clin.* 2007;25:717-740,vi.

[117] Lammie Ga, Bramman F, Wadlaw JM. Incomplite lacunar infarction (type 1b lacunes). *Acta Neuropathol.* (Berl)1998;96:163-171.

[118] Boiten J, Lodder J, Kessels F. The clinical distinct lacunar infarcts entities? *Stroke* 1993;24:652-656.

[119] Erkinjuntti T, Inzitari D, Pantoni I. et al. *J. Neurol. Trans. Suppl.* 2000;59:23-30.

[120] Van Zagten M, Lodder J, Kessels F. Gait disorders and parkinsonian signs in patients with stroke related tom small deep infarcts with matter lesions. *Mov. Disord.* 1998;13:89-95.

[121] Alarcon F, Andrade M, Rivera J. Post –stroke hemiballismus and Contralateral Tremor. Report of two cases. *Rev. Ecuat. Neurol.* 2006;15:124-126.

[122] Della Sala S. Gait apraxia by bilateral lesion of the supplementary motor area. *J. Neurol. Neurosurg. Pychiatry* 2002;72:77-85.

[123] Nakane M, Teraoka A, Asato R, Tamura A. Degeneration of the ipsilateral substantia nigra following cerebral infarction in the striatum. *Stroke* 1992;23: 328-332.

[124] Tohgi B, Utsugisawa K, Nagane Y, Mihara M. Alterations with aging and ischemia in nicotinic acetylcholine receptors subunits alpha 4 and beta 2 messenger RNA expression in postmortem human putamen. Implications for susceptibility to parkinsonism. *Brain Res.* 1998;791:186-190

[125] Mengesdorf, Jensen PH, Mies G, Paschen W. Down regulation of parkin protein in transient focal cerebral ischemia: A link between stroke and degenerative disease? *Proc. Natl. Acad. Sci. USA* 2002; 99:15042-15047.

[126] Benaroch EE. Pedunculopontino nucleus: functional organization and clinical implication. *Neurology* 2013;80:1148-1155.

[127] Fling BW, Cohen RG, Mancini M, Nutt JG, Fair DA, Horak FB. Asymmetric pedunculopontine network connectivity in parkinsonian patients with frezzing of gait. *Brain* 2013;136:2405-2418.

[128] Dubois B, Pillon B, De Saxce H, Lhermitte F, Agid Y Didsappearance of parkinsonism signs after spontaneous vascular thalamotomy. *Arch. Neurol.* 1986;43:815-817.

[129] Krauss JK, Grossman RG, Jankovic J. Improvement of parkinsonian signs after vascular lesions of the basal ganglia circuitry. *Mov. Disor.* 1997;12:124-126.

[130] Rivest J, Quinn N, Gibbs J, Marsden CD. Unilateral abolition of extrapyramidal rigidity after ipsilateral cerebellar infarction. *Mov. Disor.* 1990;5:328-330.

[131] Gouw AA, van der Flier WM, Pantoni L, Inzitari D, et al. On the Etiology of Incident Brain Lacunes: Longitudinal Observation from the LADIS Study. *Stroke* 2008; 39: 3083-3085.

[132] De Laat KF, Tuladhar AM, van Norden AGW, Norris DG,et al. Loss of white matter integrity is associated with gait disorders in cerebral small vessel disease. *Brain* 2011;134:73-83.

[133] Turinbuli Ch. Vascular Parkinsonism an important update. *Age and Ageing* 2005; 34: 97-98.

In: Parkinsonism
Editor: Cynthia Fisher
ISBN: 978-1-63483-865-8

Chapter 2

SURGICAL AND MEDICAL TREATMENT FOR NORMAL PRESSURE HYDROCEPHALUS ASSOCIATED WITH PARKINSONISM

Morgan Broggi[1,*]***, MD, PhD,***
Giovanni Tringali[1]***, MD,***
Luigi Romito[2]***, MD, Veronica Redaelli***[2]***, MD,***
Francesco Restelli[1]***, MD,***
Francesco Acerbi[1]***, MD, PhD,***
Giovanni Broggi[1]***, MD***
and Angelo Franzini[1]***, MD***

[1] Department of Neurosurgery, Fondazione IRCCS Istituto Neurologico Carlo Besta, Milano, Italy
[2] Department of Neurology, Fondazione IRCCS Istituto Neurologico Carlo Besta, Milano, Italy

* Corresponding Author: Morgan Broggi; Department of Neurosurgery, Fondazione IRCCS Istituto Neurologico Carlo Besta; Via Celoria, 11; 20133 Milano, Italy; Phone: + 39 02 23942411; Fax: + 39 02 70635017; e-mail: morganbroggi@hotmail.com

Abstract

Objective: Idiopathic normal pressure hydrocephalus (iNPH) patients may present, besides the classic triad of symptoms, extrapiramidal parkinsonian like movement disorders. We present a single blind randomized phase II study comparing surgical intervention with adjustable ventriculo-peritoneal (VP) shunt plus dopamine oral therapy (group A) versus surgical operation alone (group B) in patients affected by iNPH associated with parkinsonism.

Methods: A detailed screening process included neurological, neurosurgical and neuropsychological evaluations, followed by cerebrospinal fluid (CSF) tap test (TT), resistance outflow (Ro) measurement and CSF neurodegenerative proteins dosage. Outcome was evaluated through the Japanese NPH grading scale-revised (JNPHGSR) and the third section of the Unified Parkinson's Disease Rating Scale (UPDRS).

Results: 54 patients were screened in 36 months; 32/54 (59%) patients (mean age 73.2, range 61-80) met the inclusion criteria, but only 30 were enrolled in the study, since two patients refused to undergo surgery. 15 patients were randomized in group A and 15 in group B. Preoperative 123I-Ioflupane-cerebral SPECT (DaTSCAN) revealed some striatal dopaminergic deficit in 14/30 patients (46.5%). At the final scheduled 12 months follow-up, 23/30 patients (77% overall, 13 from group A and 10 from group B) showed an improvement of the JNPHGRS score; 19/30 patients (63% overall), 12/15 patients of group A (80%) and 7/15 patients of group B (47%), showed an improvement greater than 30% in the motor UPDRS score.

Conclusion: An association between iNPH and parkinsonism may be present in more than half of patients. In these cases, patients may benefit from VP shunt plus dopamine oral therapy.

Keywords: Cerebro-spinal fluid, DaTSCAN, normal pressure hydrocephalus, parkinsonism, ventriculo-peritoneal shunt, UPDRS

Abbreviations

CSF	cerebro spinal fluid
CT	computer tomography
DaT	dopamine transporter
DaTSCAN	123I-Ioflupane-cerebral SPECT
FAB	Frontal Assessment Battery

FDA	Food and Drug Administration
GA	general anesthesia
H-Y score	Hoehn-Yahr score
ICP	intracranial pressure
iNPH	Idiopathic normal pressure hydrocephalus
JNPHGSR	Japanese NPH grading scale-revised
MMSE	Mini Mental State Examination
MODA	Milan Overall Dementia Assessment
MR	magnetic resonance
Ro	determination of outflow Resistance
SPECT	Single photon emission computerized tomography
TT	tap test
TUG	Timed up and go test
UPDRS	Unified Parkinson's Disease Rating Scale
VP shunt	venticulo-peritoneal shunt

INTRODUCTION

Life expectancy has increased incredibly in the last 50 years in developed countries. This was a great achievement of medicine and health care systems, but at the same time, it represents a critical issue for 21st century physicians: the percentage of elderly patients is constantly increasing and consequently neurodegenerative diseases incidence [1]. Hence, neurologists and neurosurgeons are facing more and more patients affected by age related diseases.

Idiopathic normal pressure hydrocephalus (iNPH) is a potentially treatable neurological disorder of older adults that comprises disturbances of gait and balance, control of micturition, and cognition (so-called "classic triad" of symptoms of the disease) in combination with enlargement of the cerebral ventricles [2]. Gait and balance disturbances are the most common presenting findings and may occur alone or together with cognitive and urinary symptoms [2, 3, 4]. Diagnosis is often challenging due to its varied presentation and overlap with other disorders common in the elderly such as cerebrovascular and neurodegenerative diseases, urologic dysfunctions, lumbar stenosis, et cetera [5, 6]. Today, the most common treatment offered to patients is surgical shunting with venticulo-peritoneal shunt (VP shunt) [7, 8] with programmable valves [9].

Furthermore, not all patients do show the "classic triad" of symptoms; indeed, an undeniable number of patients often present signs of movement disorders, such as parkinsonism [10-12]. Diagnosis and treatment become rather challenging in this group of patients and adequate management requires both the neurologist and the neurosurgeon [13]. Up until now, they may be treated surgically with VP shunt placement or with L-dopa medications; however, there is a conspicuous lack of information concerning outcome and, more important, the proper therapy [5, 8, 14].

The incidence of this association is not clear, varying from 10% to 70% of cases in previous reports [12, 14]. It is reasonable to affirm that this condition is probably underestimated since the diagnosis, as mentioned above, is sometimes difficult and requires two skilled specialists.

The pathophysiology of parkinsonian symptoms in iNPH has not been conclusively understood. The abnormal pulsation of cerebro spinal fluid (CSF) flow occurring in hydrocephalus may produce a secondary damage to the nigrostriatal dopaminergic pathway and a down regulation of D2 receptors in the striatum and putamen [15-17]. Moreover, the meso-limbic dopaminergic pathway and the ascending reticular activating system may also be injured in some cases of severe and longstanding iNPH [14].

Single photon emission computerized tomography (SPECT) of the dopamine transporter (DaT), a marker of nigrostriatal degeneration, is a recent advance in imaging that supports the clinician in the differential diagnosis of movement disorders [18-22]; this technique is known as (123I-Ioflupane) SPECT or, more simply, DaTSCAN [23].

In such a scenario, CSF biomarkers, that reflect the ongoing pathophysiological process, might further help the comprehension of iNPH or other neurodegenerative diseases biological mechanisms [24-28].

We designed a study aiming at better clarifying the actual incidence of the association iNPH-parkinsonism and at comparing the clinical outcome between VP shunt alone and VP shunt plus oral dopaminergic therapy for patients affected by the aforementioned association.

Materials and Methods

Study Design and Inclusion/Exclusion Criteria

This is a prospective a single blind randomized phase II study comparing surgical intervention with adjustable VP shunt plus dopamine oral therapy (group A) versus surgical operation alone (group B) in patients affected by iNPH associated with parkinsonism. The study lasted 48 months.

Inclusion criteria were as follows: a) age between 60 and 80. b) Beginning of symptoms at least 6 months before. c) Diagnosis of iNPH associated with parkinsonism made cooperatively by a neurosurgeon and a neurologist at the end of a detailed screening process (described below). d) third (motor) section of the Unified Parkinson's Disease Rating Scale (UPDRS) between 15 and 50 and Hoehn-Yahr (H-Y score) between 1 and 3.

Exclusion criteria were as follows: a) preexisting diagnosis of neurodegenerative diseases (e.g., Parkinson or Alzheimer disease, vascular dementia). b) pre-existing diagnosis of malignant cancer of any type. c) pre-existing diagnosis of psychiatric disease with use of drugs that may interfere with dopaminergic medications. d) pre-existing diagnosis of bowel malabsorption syndrome that may interfere or compromise dopaminergic medications effects. e) previous head or abdominal surgeries of any type. f) inability to undergo computer tomography (CT) scan, magnetic resonance (MR) scan, general anesthesia (GA) or to give informed consent for any reason.

Diagnosis and Enrollment

These were made by 2 steps: a) clinical and radiological evaluation of the patient during outpatient clinics either by the neurosurgeon or by the neurologist with suspect of iNPH associated to parkinsoninsm. b) Step two consisted of a short hospital admission (usually 24-48 hours) during which: first, diagnosis of iNPH had to be confirmed through close clinical assessment, review or, if needed, execution of radiological exams (Figure 1) and calculation of Japanese NPH grading scale-revised (JNPHGSR) [14] (Table 1), and invasive CSF tests (intracranial pressure (ICP) measurement, tap test (TT) and determination of outflow Resistance, (Ro)), according to previous published guidelines [5]; second, parkinsonism had to be validated by the neurologist along with calculation of baseline third section of the UPDRS (Table 2) according to inclusion criteria (see above); and third, neurocognitive tests (e.g., Mini Mental State Examination (MMSE) [29], Frontal Assessment Battery (FAB) [30-31], Milan Overall Dementia Assessment (MODA) [32], Tinetti's Scale [33], Timed up and go test (TUG) [34] were carried out as well in order to exclude patients affected by other neurodegenerative disorders (e.g., Parkinson or Alzheimer disease, vascular dementia, et cetera).

Table 1. Japanese NPH grading scale-revised (from reference no. 14, *see text*)

Score	**gait disturbances**	**cognitive disturbances**	**urinary disturbances**
0	normal	normal	normal
1	dizziness, or awareness of gait disturbance	awareness of attention and memory disturbance	pollakisuria, or urinary urgency
2	gait disturbance (not requiring aid)	Impaired attention and memory (not disoriented)	occasional incontinence (more than 1–3/week)
3	inability to walk without aid (stick, hand-rail, or walker)	continuous disorientation of time and place	frequent incontinence (more than 1/day)
4	Complete inability to walk	severe, continuous disorientation and/or loss of verbal ability	almost total loss of bladder control

Table 2. III section (motor examination) of the UPDRS, items from 18 to 31

18. Speech	
0	Normal
1	Slight loss of expression, diction and/or volume
2	Monotone, slurred but understandable; moderately impaired
3	Marked impairment, difficult to understand
4	Unintelligible
19. Facial Expression	
0	Normal
1	Minimal hypomimia, could be normal "Poker Face"
2	Slight but definitely abnormal diminution of facial expression
3	Moderate hypomimia; lips parted some of the time
4	Masked or fixed facies with severe or complete loss of facial expression; lips parted 1/4 inch or more
20. Tremor at rest (head, upper and lower extremities)	
0	Absent
1	Slight and infrequently present
2	Mild in amplitude and persistent. Or moderate in amplitude, but only intermittently present
3	Moderate in amplitude and present most of the time

4	Marked in amplitude and present most of the time
21. Action or Postural Tremor of hands	
0	Absent
1	Slight; present with action
2	Moderate in amplitude, present with action
3	Moderate in amplitude with posture holding as well as action
4	Marked in amplitude; interferes with feeding
22. Rigidity (Judged on passive movement of major joints with patient relaxed in sitting position. Cogwheeling to be ignored.)	
0	Absent
1	Slight or detectable only when activated by mirror or other movements
2	Mild to moderate
3	Marked, but full range of motion easily achieved
4	Severe, range of motion achieved with difficulty
23. Finger Taps (Patient taps thumb with index finger in rapid succession.)	
0	Normal
1	Mild slowing and/or reduction in amplitude
2	Moderately impaired. Definite and early fatiguing. May have occasional arrests in movement
3	Severely impaired. Frequent hesitation in initiating movements or arrests in ongoing movement
4	Can barely perform the task
24. Hand Movements (Patient opens and closes hands in rapid succesion.)	
0	Normal
1	Mild slowing and/or reduction in amplitude
2	Moderately impaired. Definite and early fatiguing. May have occasional arrests in movement
3	Severely impaired. Frequent hesitation in initiating movements or arrests in ongoing movement
4	Can barely perform the task
25. Rapid Alternating Movements of Hands (Pronation-supination movements of hands, vertically and horizontally, with as large an amplitude as possible, both hands simultaneously.)	
0	Normal
1	Mild slowing and/or reduction in amplitude
2	Moderately impaired. Definite and early fatiguing. May have occasional arrests in movement
3	Severely impaired. Frequent hesitation in initiating movements or arrests in ongoing movement
4	Can barely perform the task

Table 2. (Continued)

26. Leg Agility (Patient taps heel on the ground in rapid succession picking up entire leg. Amplitude should be at least 3 inches.)	
0	Normal
1	Mild slowing and/or reduction in amplitude
2	Moderately impaired. Definite and early fatiguing. May have occasional arrests in movement
3	Severely impaired. Frequent hesitation in initiating movements or arrests in ongoing movement
4	Can barely perform the task
27. Arising from Chair. (Patient attempts to rise from a straightbacked chair, with arms folded across chest.)	
0	Normal
1	Slow; or may need more than one attempt
2	Pushes self up from arms of seat
3	Tends to fall back and may have to try more than one time, but can get up without help.
4	Unable to arise without help
28. Posture	
0	Normal erect
1	Not quite erect, slightly stooped posture; could be normal for older person
2	Moderately stooped posture, definitely abnormal; can be slightly leaning to one side
3	Severely stooped posture with kyphosis; can be moderately leaning to one side
4	Marked flexion with extreme abnormality of posture
29. Gait	
0	Normal
1	Walks slowly, may shuffle with short steps, but no festination (hastening steps) or propulsion
2	Walks with difficulty, but requires little or no assistance; may have some festination, short steps, or propulsion
3	Severe disturbance of gait, requiring assistance
4	Cannot walk at all, even with assistance
30. Postural Stability (Response to sudden, strong posterior displacement produced by pull on shoulders while patient erect with eyes open and feet slightly apart. Patient is prepared.)	
0	Normal
1	Retropulsion, but recovers unaided
2	Absence of postural response; would fall if not caught by examiner
3	Very unstable, tends to lose balance spontaneously

4	Unable to stand without assistance
31. Body Bradykinesia and Hypokinesia (Combining slowness, hesitancy, decreased armswing, small amplitude, and poverty of movement in general.)	
0	None
1	Minimal slowness, giving movement a deliberate character; could be normal for some persons. Possibly reduced amplitude.
2	Mild degree of slowness and poverty of movement which is definitely abnormal. Alternatively, some reduced amplitude.
3	Moderate slowness, poverty or small amplitude of movement.
4	Marked slowness, poverty or small amplitude of movement

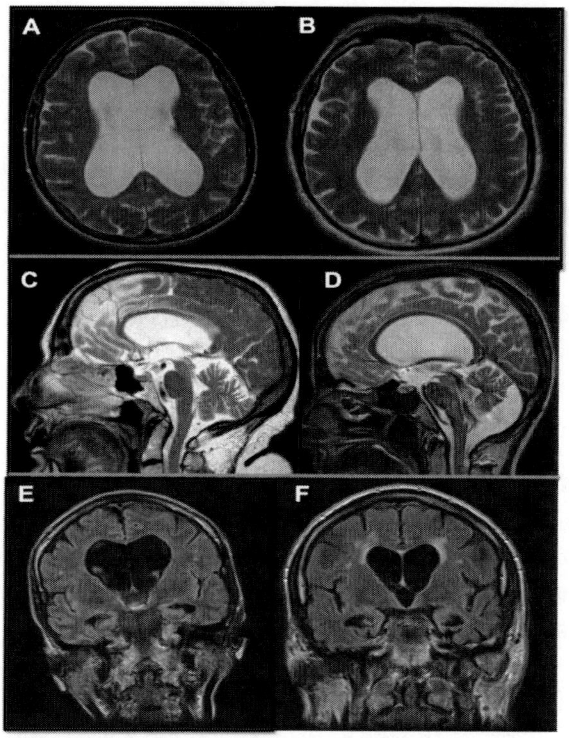

Figure 1. Preoperative MR images of patients included in the study. A and B are axial T-2 weighted. C and D are sagittal T-2 weighted; note how the corpus callosum is stretched by the hydrocephalus, especially in D. E and F are coronal FLAIR images; note the mild transependimal CSF reabrorption, especially in F.

At this stage patients were enrolled in the study, signed the informed consent and were randomized into group A or B (see above). They were discharged and were scheduled for 123I-Ioflupane-cerebral SPECT (DaTSCAN) as an outpatient and for VP shunt within 4 months from enrollment (see below).

DaTSCAN was evaluated as follows: i) grade 0: normal largely symmetrical in putamen and caudate; ii) grade 1: asymmetrically reduced putamen/caudate activity; iii) grade 2: significant bilaterally reduced putamen/caudate uptake; iv) grade 3: virtually absent uptake bilaterally affecting both putamen and caudate nuclei.

Surgical Procedure and Follow-up

A new hospital admission was organized within 4 months from enrollment: at admission clinical examination and cognitive tests were repeated: patients who showed a significant cognitive deterioration (more than 5 points at MMSE) from enrollment were excluded. Conversely, those with stable cognitive deficit underwent VP shunt.

VP shunt operation was performed in a standardized way: under GA, through a pre-coronal burr hole (usually right side) a ventricular catheter was positioned (Figure 2) and then connected to an adjustable valve (Codman-Hakim programmable valve, Codman Johnson&Johnson company, Raynham, MA, USA) and to a distal catheter that was introduced into the peritoneum running under the skin. The valve was initially regulated based on the preoperative TT and Ro, usually between 120 and 150 mmH2O.

During VP shunt operation, CSF was collected and sent for t-tau, p-tau-181 and Aβ42 proteins dosage. Within 72 hours from surgery, after having excluded acute surgical complications (hemorrhage, catheters wrong placement, et cetera) group A patients began oral therapy with Levodopa/Carbidopa 100+25 mg 1+1/2 tablet 4 times daily. During the whole course of the study, patients were not allowed to assume other medications with dopaminergic or antidopaminergic activity; if these drugs would be necessary (e.g., development of psychotic disorders), the patient was excluded.

The follow-up was planned to last 12 months, with visits (both neurological and neurosurgical) every 3 months (i.e., 4 visit total) during which valve or Levodopa/Carbidopa dosage adjustments could be possible. The visits always comprised neurological examination with calculation of motor section of the UPDRS.

Dosage of CSF proteins was repeated once during the whole follow-up, at third visit (nine months after VP shunt). Last calculation of motor section of the UPDRS was done by a different neurologist blinded as to the type of treatment administered and instructed not to investigate it. Patients were instructed as well not to give information about treatment. After 12 months from VP shunt, further follow-up visits (no more evaluated in the study) were scheduled yearly, unless the patient complained new symptoms or rapid worsening of pre-existing ones.

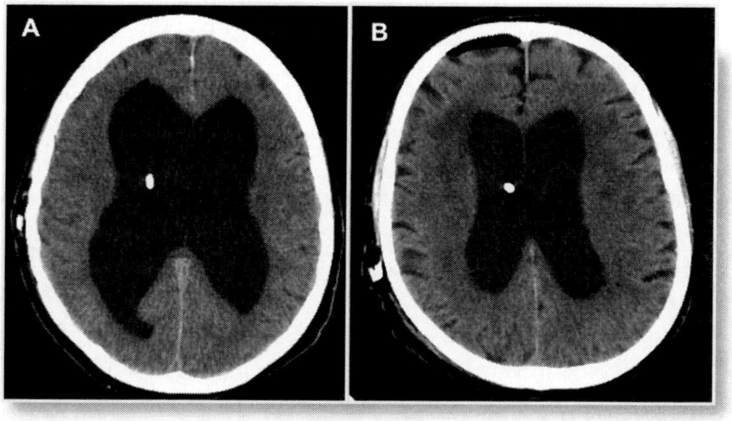

Figure 2. A and B Postoperative images after VP shunt with the ventricular catheter inserted into the righ lateral ventricle through a right precoronal burr hole access.

Outcome Evaluation

The primary endpoint was the proportion of patients in the two groups with an improvement greater than 30% in the motor section of the UPDRS between the baseline and the 12 months follow-up; this value was chosen based on the threshold considered significant for the acute Levodopa challenge [35].

The secondary endpoints comprised: i) the evaluation of the clinical outcome calculated through the JNPHGSR and the neuropsychological tests (MMSE, FAB, MODA, Tinetti's Scale, TUG) between the baseline and the 12 months follow-up; ii) the value of baseline DaTSCAN in predicting the clinical outcome the motor outocome (primary endpoint) correlating its baseline grade (from 0 to 3) and; iii) the analysis of degenerative CSF proteins, evaluating the variations of their concentration in the CSF between the baseline and the follow-up and therefore if this could be influenced by the treatment.

RESULTS

Enrollment and Surgery

In the screening phase that lasted 36 months, 54 patients were considered suitable for the study either by neurosurgeons or by neurologists and were admitted to the hospital to confirm enrollment. 22/54 (41%) patients were not included in the study for the following reasons: 6 patients (11% overall, 27% of the excluded) had a good response to the TT and positive Ro measurement, but were excluded by the neurologist for not being affected by parkinsonism; anyway, these patients were treated with VP shunt. Another 8 patients (15% overall, 36% of the excluded) did not show any an improvement of their symptoms with the TT; none of these were treated surgically. 3 patients (5% overall, 13% of the excluded) showed only slight improvement after TT and had a negative measurement of Ro and they were not treated surgically, while 2 patients (4% overall, 9% of the excluded) showed only slight improvement after TT, but had a positive measurement of Ro and underwent VP shunt. Some of these patients received dopaminergic medications too. Finally, 3 patients (5% overall, 13% of the excluded) were excluded either due to a very compromised cognitive status without significant motor deficit or because they were not judged suitable to undergo GA.

On the other hand, 32/54 (59%) patients (mean age 73.2, range 61-80; 17 males and 13 females with a M:F ratio 1.3;) met the inclusion criteria, were diagnosed as being affected by iNPH and parkinsonism and were enrolled in the study.

Actually only 30/54 patients (55%) were finally included in the study, since two patients refused to undergo surgery. Therefore, 15 patients were randomized in group A and 15 in group B.

Pretreatment data on these 30 patients are summarized in Table 3 and 4.

Table 3. Datailed pretreatment data of the 30 patients included in the study

Pt.	Gr.	J NPH GSR	UP DRS	H-Y	MMSE	FAB	MODA	Tinetti	TUG	J NPH GRS post TT	Aβ42	p-tau-181	t-tau
1	A	8	24	2,5	24	16	86	19	14,75	6	394	55	785
2	A	6	22	3	27,5	18	91	21	15,51	5	945	50	128
3	B	4	25	3	30	17	98,2	19	15,23	3	358	53	379
4	A	7	25	2,5	25,3	15	72,7	15	21,24	5	392	24	893
5	B	4	29	3	27	18	90	19	18,85	3	473	47	634
6	A	5	32	3	25	11	77	9	27,64	4	624	44	345
7	A	8	26	3	25	15	83,3	10	29,98	6	582	26	193
8	B	7	28	2,5	25,3	9,2	82	11	36,37	6	692	54	299
9	B	9	33	2	23,4	9	78	8	32,75	6	826	19	129
10	B	5	24	3	30	16	93,3	16	27,34	4	450	46	185
11	A	8	28	2,5	23,7	15	90,5	15	26,1	5	690	23	285
12	A	6	22	3	27,3	17	88	14	24,3	5	286	57	751
13	A	4	29	3	26	9,2	73,3	11	24,2	4	352	20	135
14	B	6	27	3	25,5	17	92,7	20	18,9	5	589	53	395
15	B	7	31	2	24,5	10	73,5	16	25,69	5	852	59	402
16	B	5	32	3	24,5	8	75	18	26,63	4	1045	29	189
17	B	4	23	3	28,3	18	92,7	22	16,5	4	679	34	359
18	A	6	27	3	30	14	86,9	19	20,09	4	669	27	117
19	B	9	24	2,5	23,4	15,3	85,5	22	15,53	6	1071	24	166
20	A	7	25	3	25	14,5	82,5	17	14,61	6	575	22	85

Pt.	Gr.	J NPH GSR	UP DRS	H-Y	MMSE	FAB	MODA	Tinetti	TUG	J NPH GRS post TT	Aβ42	p-tau-181	t-tau
21	A	5	29	3	26	18	93,7	18	17,65	3	1159	82	747
22	A	6	29	3	27,3	14	86,5	19	18,51	4	497	46	884
23	B	7	21	2	23,3	14	76,5	16	19,89	5	683	26	160
24	B	5	27	3	27	15	93,5	18	20,25	3	678	45	254
25	A	5	34	3	26,86	13	82,5	6	36,43	3	308	23	121
26	A	6	23	2	24,5	17	93,7	15	25,28	5	635	20	101
27	B	8	34	3	26,5	8,5	73	5	57,64	7	373	235	355
28	B	4	24	2,5	26	17,4	97	18	14,73	3	213	47	1161
29	A	5	30	3	29	17	91,3	13	20,28	4	276	26	155
30	B	4	25	3	24,7	17,2	90,8	18	14,25	3	686	49	614

Legend:

Pt.: patient number; Gr.: group of randomization; JNPHGSR: Japanese NPH grading scale-revised; UPDRS: Unified Parkinson's Disease Rating Scale; H-Y: Hoehn-Yahr score; MMSE: Mini Mental State Examination; FAB: Frontal Assesment Battery; MODA: Milan Overall Dementia Assessment; Tinetti: Tinetti's scale; TUG: Timed up and go test; TT: tap test. t-tau, p-tau-181 and Aβ42 dosage are in pg/ml.

Table 4. Summary of pretreatment data of the 30 patients included in the study

Demographic data	**Mean values**	**range**
Age	73.2	61-80
M:F ratio	1.3	17 M; 13 F
Scale		
JNPHGSR	6/12	4-9
UPDRS	27,07/108	21-34
H-Y score	2,77/5	2-3
MMSE	26,06/30	23,3-30
FAB	14,44/18	8-18
MODA	85,69/100	72,7-98,2
Tinetti's scale	15,57/28	5-22
TUG	23,24 sec	14,25-57,64 sec
JNPHGRS post TT	4,53/12	3-7
CSF neurodegenerative proteins dosage		
t-tau (pg/ml)	380,2	85-1161
p-tau-181 (pg/ml)	45,5	19-235
Aβ42 (pg/ml)	601,73	213-1159

Legend:

M: Males; F: Females; JNPHGSR: Japanese NPH grading scale-revised; UPDRS: Unified Parkinson's Disease Rating Scale; H-Y score: Hoehn-Yahr score; MMSE: Mini Mental State Examination; FAB: Frontal Assesment Battery; MODA: Milan Overall Dementia Assessment; TUG: Timed up and go test; TT: tap test.

In details, mean JNPHGRS was 6/12 (range 4-9), while mean third section UPDRS was 27.07/108 (range 21-34) and H-Y score 2.77 (range 2-3).

Concerning the cognitive tests, their preoperative mean values were as follows:

- MMSE: 26.06 (range 23.3-30)
- FAB: 14.44 (range 8-18)
- MODA: 85.69 (range 72.7-98.2)
- Tinetti's Scale: 15.57 (range 5-22)
- TUG: 23.24 seconds (range 14.25-57.64)

Mean JNPHGRS after TT was 4.53 (range 3-7).

Preoperative DaTSCAN revealed some striatal dopaminergic deficit in 14/30 patients (46.5%) (Figure 3), 7 in both group A and B. Specifically, there were no grade 3 DaTSCAN, while there were 5 grade 2 (3 in group A and 2 in group B) and 9 grade 1 DaTSCAN (4 in group A and 5 in group B)

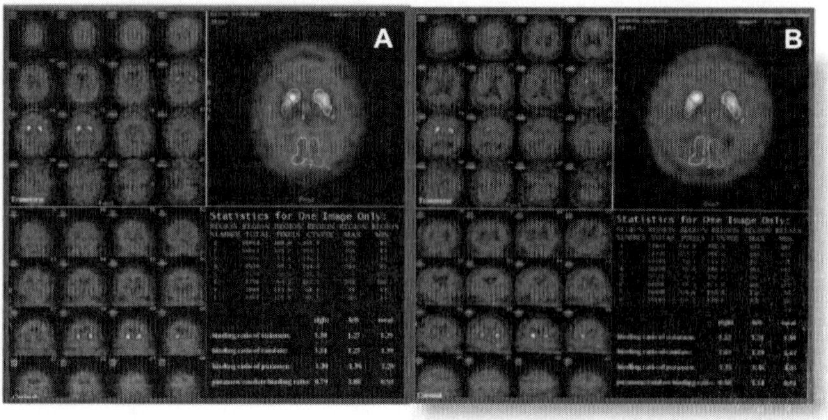

Figure 3. Two examples of grade 1 postive DaTSCAN.

The dosage of CSF protein obtained during VP shunt operation were as follows:

- t-tau: 380.20 pg/ml (normal range 60-70 y.o. < 400 pg/ml; 70-80 y.o. < 500 pg/ml) with a range of 85-1161 pg/ml.
- p-tau-181: 45.50 pg/ml (normal range < 61 pg/ml) with a range of 19-235 pg/ml.
- Aβ42: 601.73 pg/ml (normal range > 500 pg/ml) with a normal range of 213-1159 pg/ml.

Surgical mortality was 0%. Complications related to VP shunt were as follows: VP shunt infection 0%; VP shunt malfunction 0%; abdominal complication (infection and peritonitis, bowel perforation, et cetera) 0%; intracerebral hematoma (not requiring surgical drainage) causing seizure and slight monoparesis (arm and hand, not requiring rehabilitation) 1 case (3%); ventricular catheter displacement that required repositioning, 1 case (3%); abdominal catheter displacement that required repositioning, 2 cases (7%); igromas due to hyperdrainage (not requiring surgical drainage, but only valve adjustments), 3 cases (10%).

Surgical complications are summarized in Table 5.

Table 5. Complication rate related to VP shunt in the current series

Complications	n. of patients	overall percentage
mortality	0	0%
VP shunt infection	0	0%
VP shunt malfunction	0	0%
Abdominal complication	0	0%
Intracerebral hematoma	1	3%
Ventricular catheter displacement	1	3%
Abdominal catheter displacement	2	7%
Igromas due to hyperdrainage	3	10%

Legend:
VP shunt: Ventriculo-peritoneal shunt

Follow-up and Outcome Evaluation

All patients completed the entire follow-up program of 12 months (4 visits, one every 3 months). At last follow-up of 12 months, 23/30 patients (77% overall, 13 from group A and 10 from group B) showed an improvement of the JNPHGRS score; 19/30 patients (63% overall), 12/15 patients of group A (80%) and 7/15 (47%) patients of group B, showed an improvement greater than 30% in the UPDRS score. Of the 3 patients in group A that did not achieve the >30% UDPRS improvement, 2 had a grade 2 positive DaTSCAN and one a grade 1, while of the 8 patients that did not achieve the >30% UDPRS improvement, 2 had a grade 2 positive DaTSCAN, 3 had a grade 1 and 3 had a negative DaTSCAN. Conversely, 1 group A patient with a grade 2 and 3 with a grade 1 positive DaTSCAN reached the >30% UDPRS improvement, while 2 group B patient with grade 1 positive DaTSCAN reached the >30% UDPRS improvement.

Outcome data at 12 months of follow-up are summarized in Table 6 and 7.

Table 6. Detailed outcome data (12 months follow-up) of the 30 patients included in the study

Pt.	Gr.	JNPH GSR	UPDRS	MMSE	FAB	MODA	Tinetti	TUG	Aβ42	p-tau-181	t-tau
1	A	5	16	27	17	93	27	12,65	978	92	788
2	A	4	17	27	18	97,7	28	13,1	673	63	372
3	B	4	16	30	18	98,2	27	12,43	299	61	220
4	A	5	17	29	16	85,5	22	24,56	276	45	128
5	B	4	20	27	17	95,7	26	17,12	855	34	122
6	A	2	22	28	14	86,3	14	24,78	515	67	274
7	A	5	17	29	16	94,3	18	34,73	469	39	160
8	B	7	19	26,5	12,5	92	26	27,5	695	122	862
9	B	6	22	24	11,5	88,3	14	25,23	935	38	122
10	B	2	23	30	15	97	21	21,22	379	49	192
11	A	4	26	26	17	96,3	19	22,35	948	44	180
12	A	4	20	28,5	18	93,5	18	21,79	853	94	192
13	A	1	19	28	13	82,3	18	22,33	299	63	483
14	B	3	16	26,5	18	95,5	24	15,89	677	97	655
15	B	4	20	27	14	80	18	18,1	634	88	792
16	B	3	22	26	13	85	26	21,98	1079	67	390
17	B	2	15	29	18	90	23	14,9	893	55	239
18	A	3	24	30	18	91	23	15,33	345	18	167
19	B	4	23	21,3	11,3	74,7	28	15,69	1168	65	425
20	A	8	23	27	16	84	25	16,32	1166	62	337

Pt.	Gr.	JNPH GSR	UPDRS	MMSE	FAB	MODA	Tinetti	TUG	Aβ42	p-tau-181	t-tau
21	A	4	15	30	18	98	25	15,24	1123	135	932
22	A	6	25	28,5	16	89	23	15,5	790	37	178
23	B	7	20	25	15	82	24	12,34	795	65	534
24	B	1	30	28	17	88	26	11,39	563	84	623
25	A	4	23	30	17	92	21	18,9	481	35	172
26	A	4	25	29	18	95	12	28,61	467	14	86
27	B	3	22	28,5	15,7	87	17	37,86	982	67	295
28	B	1	15	28,47	16,3	95,2	23	13,18	798	31	123
29	A	4	19	30	18	98	19	25,45	499	164	1008
30	B	4	16	23,2	18	90,4	28	11,48	535	80	353

Legend:

Pt.: patient number; Gr.: group of randomization; JNPHGSR: Japanese NPH grading scale-revised; UPDRS: Unified Parkinson's Disease Rating Scale; H-Y: Hoehn-Yahr score; MMSE: Mini Mental State Examination; FAB: Frontal Assesment Battery; MODA: Milan Overall Dementia Assessment; Tinetti: Tinetti's scale; TUG: Timed up and go test; TT: tap test. t-tau, p-tau-181 and Aβ42 dosage are in pg/ml.

Table 7. Summary of outcome data (12 months follow-up) of the 30 patients included in the study

Scales	**values**	**range**
JNPHGRS	3,93/12	1-8
UPDRS	20,23/108	15-30
MMSE	27,58/30	21,3-30
FAB	16,01/18	11,3-18
MODA	90,50/100	74,7-98,2
Tinetti's scale	22,10/28	12-28
TUG	19,60 s	11,39-37,86
CSF neurodegenerative proteins dosage		
t-tau (pg/ml)	380,13	86-1008
p-tau-181 (pg/ml)	65,83	14-164
Aβ42 (pg/ml)	705,63	276-1168

Legend:

JNPHGSR: Japanese NPH grading scale-revised; UPDRS: Unified Parkinson's Disease Rating Scale; MMSE: Mini Mental State Examination; FAB: Frontal Assesment Battery; MODA: Milan Overall Dementia Assessment; TUG: Timed up and go test.

In details, mean JNPHGRS was 3.93/12 (range 1-8), while mean UPDRS (third section) was 20.23/108 (range 15-30).

Concerning the cognitive tests, their mean values were as follows:

- MMSE: 27.58 (range 21.3-30)
- FAB: 16.01 (range 11.3-18)
- MODA: 90.50 (range 74.7-98.2)
- Tinetti's Scale: 22.10 (range 12-28)
- TUG: 19.60 seconds (range 11.39-37.86)

The dosage of CSF protein obtained at follow-up were as follows:

- t-tau: 380.13 pg/ml (normal range 60-70 y.o. < 400 pg/ml; 70-80 y.o. < 500 pg/ml) with a range of 86-1008 pg/ml.
- p-tau-181: 65.83 pg/ml (normal range < 61 pg/ml) with a range of 14-164 pg/ml.
- Aβ42: 705.63 pg/ml (normal range > 500 pg/ml) with a normal range of 276-1168 pg/ml.

Discussion

The so-called "ageing population" is a well-known phenomenon of the 21st century. Of course, the increased life expectancy of the population is a concrete achievement of our times, but, indeed, it deserves to be critically evaluated since it represents a great challenge for the next future: people aged over 65 will double from 11% of the whole population to 22% in 2050 [1]. As a consequence, neurologists and neurosurgeons are facing more and more patients affected by (age related) neurodegenerative diseases.

iNPH is a condition characterized by ventricular enlargement and normal ICP caused by disturbed CSF dynamics [2]. The initial presentation includes a slowly progressive impairment of gait and balance, cognitive deterioration and urinary incontinence, also known as "classic triad" [5].

The condition may be treated by means of a shunt that drains the excess of CFS in another part of the body; today, the most common shunt used is the VP shunt [7, 8] with programmable valves [9]. The results of shunt implantation in iNPH patients are good, with an improvement rate of more than 80% in recent studies [36, 37] and the complication rate is fairly low [38]. The cause of the disease is still unknown [39].

Rather often iNPH symptoms may overlap with other disorders common in the elderly and the "classic triad" may not be clearly evident [5, 6]. In particular patients may preset many different movement disorders, but the most common are extrapyramidal parkinsonian like symptoms [10-12]. The pathogenesis is unclear too. The exact incidence of this association is not known. Some authors do not even report any case of such a relationship, while others describe parkinsonian symptoms in iNPH patients in a range between 11% and 70% of cases [12, 14]. It seems reasonable however, that, due to its insidious presentation that requires both the neurologist and the neurosurgeon [13]), it is underestimated.

Therefore, when approaching patients with these characteristic a truly complete diagnostic flowchart should be recommended, including DaTSCAN and CSF degenerative proteins dosage.

DaTSCAN, (123I-Ioflupane) SPECT, is a recent advance in imaging that supports the clinician in the differential diagnosis of movement disorders [18-22]. It has been demonstrated that, in vitro, ioflupane binds reversibly to human recombinant DaT and that the binding of ioflupane in the striatum is abolished by the dopamine reuptake inhibitor GBR 12909, thereby demonstrating the selectivity of ioflupane binding to striatal presynaptic DaT. DaTSCAN has been approved for use in SPECT imaging in Europe since

2000, and recently the Food and Drug Administration (FDA) has now approved it for use in the United States too [23].

Though there are several CSF proteins which were previously studied and some of these showed an association with iNPH [24-27], most of them still require further verification [28].

The present prospective study provides some interesting data. First of all, it shows that the association between iNPH and parkinsonism is rather common; in this series almost 60% of patients screened (32 out of 54) were diagnosed to harbor this association following a strict diagnostic process. These patients, that usually present a predominance of motor symptoms, should be treated by the neurologist and the neurosurgeon together [13].

Although it is already known that VP shunt may be a successful treatment for both iNPH and iNPH associated with parkinsonism [14, 36, 37], this study is the first that aims to investigate whether VP shunt plus oral dopaminergic therapy may further improve patients outcome, especially the motor deficits (primary endpoint). Indeed, similarly to previous literature data [14, 36, 37], 77% of patients showed a general improvement in their clinical status measured through the JNPHGRS, but, even more interesting 19/30 patients (63% overall) showed an improvement greater than 30% in the motor section of the UPDRS score; of these, 12 were in the group the received both VP shunt and dopaminergic drugs. All neurocognitve tests showed an improvement as well in both groups of patients after treatment (secondary endpoint).

Concerning the other two secondary endpoints (the value of baseline DaTSCAN and the analysis of degenerative CSF proteins), some considerations should be made on preoperative DaTSCAN; is baseline DaTSCAN able to predict patients' response to treatment (i.e., those whit positive pretreatment DaTSCAN will not improve?) At present we do not have a definitive answer. Anyway, we can say that it can give an overview on how compromised is the nigrostriatial system, but it has not an absolute value in predicting outcome; in this series, for example, there were 6 patients with positive DaTSCAN (one with grade 2) that reached a >30% UDPRS improvement either with VP shunt alone or with VP shunt plus oral dopaminergic therapy.

Looking at neurodenerative CSF proteins dosage, while t-tau and Aβ42 were both within normal range before and after the operation, surprisingly p-tau-181 increased to abnormal range after VP shunt. It seems therefore that t-tau and Aβ42 concentration are not influenced by treatment. Conversely affirming that the p-tau-181 CSF dosage is surely influenced by the treatment seems fairly hazardous. This is the first study that compares CSF degenerative proteins before and after VP shunt; larger studied are needed to confirm and/or to discuss these findings.

Dealing with such a particular pathology, the major limitation of the study is that it is a single center study and the patient sample is rather small. The Fondazione IRCCS Istituto Besta is a referral center in Italy for movement disorders and consequently many patients with parkinsonian like symptoms are referred to this center; this could in part explain the high percentage (59%) of cases screened found to harbor the association between iNPH and parkinsonism. Planning a multicenter study may shad more light on this disease and may lead to new advances in understanding its pathophysiology. Specifically, new stimulating data could arise concerning the role of both DaTSCAN (maybe repeating the exam also after treatment) and CFS proteins dosage.

Conclusion

Diagnosis of the association between iNPH and parkinsonism is challenging and therefore a close collaboration between the neurologist and the neurosurgeon plus a strict diagnostic protocol is recommended. Indeed, this association may be present in more than half of patients that present typical symptoms of these diseases. In these cases, patients may benefit from VP shunt plus dopamine oral therapy.

References

[1] Scafato E, Gandin C, Galluzzo L, Ghirini S, Cacciatore F, Capurso A, Solfrizzi V, Panza F, Cocchi A, Consoli D, Enzi G, Frisoni GB, Gandolfo C, Giampaoli S, Inzitari D, Maggi S, Crepaldi G, Mariotti S, Mecocci P, Motta M, Negrini R, Postacchini D, Rengo F, Farchi G; I.PR.E.A. Working Group (Italian PRoject on Epidemiology of Alzheimer's disease): Prevalence of aging-associated cognitive decline in an Italian elderly population: results from cross-sectional phase of Italian PRoject on Epidemiology of Alzheimer's disease (IPREA). *Aging Clin Exp Res* 22(5-6):440-449, 2010.

[2] Adams RD, Fisher CM, Hakim S, Ojemann RG, Sweet WH. Symptomatic occult hydrocephalus with ''normal'' cerebrospinal-fluid pressure: a treatable syndrome. *N Engl J Med* 1965;273:117-126.

[3] Ojemann RG, Fisher CM, Adams RD, Sweet WH, New PF: Further experiences with the syndrome of normal pressure hydrocephalus. *J Neurosurg* 31:279-294, 1969.

[4] McGirt MJ, Woodworth G, Coon AL, Thomas G, Williams MA, Rigamonti D. Diagnosis, treatment, and analysis of long-term outcomes in idiopathic normal-pressure hydrocephalus. *Neurosurgery* 2005;57(4):699-705.

[5] Relkin N, Marmarou A, Klinge P, Bergsneider M, Black PM. Diagnosing idiopathic normal-pressure hydrocephalus. *Neurosurgery* 2005;57(3 Suppl):S4-16.

[6] Bech-Azeddine R, Waldemar G, Knudsen GM, Hogh P, Brahn P,Wildschiodtz G, Gjerris F, Paulson OB, Juhler M: Idiopathic normal pressure hydrocephalus: Evaluation and findings in a multidisciplinary memory clinic. *Eur J Neurol* 8:601-611, 2001.

[7] Hebb AO, Cusimano MD. Idiopathic normal pressure hydrocephalus: a systematic review of diagnosis and outcome. *Neurosurgery* 2001;49:1166-1186.

[8] Tsakanikas D, Relknn N. Normal pressure hydrocephalus. *Semin Neruol* 2007;27(1):58-65.

[9] Bergsneider M, Black PM, Klinge P, et al. Surgical management of idiopathic normal-pressure hydrocephalus. *Neurosurgery* 2005;57(3 Suppl):S29-S39.

[10] Curran T, Lang AE. Parkinsonian syndromes associated with hydrocephalus: case reports, a review of the literature, and pathophysiological hypotheses. *Mov Disord* 1994;9:508-520.

[11] Ishii M, Akiguchi I. Recovery process of gait disturbance after ventriculo-peritoneal shunt in patients with idiopathic normal pressure hydrocephalus. *J Phys Ther Sci* 2007;19:183-188.

[12] Krauss JK, Regel JP, Droste DW, Orszagh M, Borremans JJ, Vach W. Movement disorders in adult hydrocephalus. *Mov Disord* 1997;12:53-60.

[13] Broggi M, Romito L, Redaelli V, Franzini A. Normal pressure hydrocephalus and parkinsonism: the essential teamwork between the neurosurgeon and the neurologist. *World Neurosurg* 2014;82(6):e837-8.

[14] Akiguchi I, Ishii M, Watanabe Y, Watanabe T, Kawasaki T, Yagi H, Shiino A, Shirakashi Y, Kawamoto Y. Shunt-responsive parkinsonism

and reversible white matter lesions in patients with idiopathic NPH. *J Neurol* 2008 Sep;255(9):1392-9.

[15] Stolze H, Kuhtz-Buschbeck JP, Drucke H, John K, Illert M, Deuschl G. Comparative analysis of the gait disorder of normal pressure hydrocephalus and Parkinson's disease. *J Neurol Neurosurg Psychiatry* 2001;70:289-297.

[16] Racette BA, Esper GJ, Antenor J, Black KJ, Burkey A, Moerlein SM, Videen TO, Kotagal V, Ojemann JG, Perlmutter JS. Pathophysiology of parkinsonism due to hydrocephalus. *J Neurol Neurosurg Psychiatry* 2004;75:1617-1619.

[17] Ouchi Y, Nakayama T, Kanno T, Yoshikawa E, Shinke T, Torizuka T. In vivo presynaptic and postsynaptic striatal dopamine functions in idiopathic normal pressure hydrocephalus. *J Cereb Blood Flow Metab* 2007;27:803-810.

[18] Catafau AM, Tolosa E. Impact of dopamine transporter SPECT using 123I-Ioflupane on diagnosis and management of patients with clinically uncertain Parkinsonian syndromes. *Mov Disord* 2004;19:1175-1182.

[19] Tolosa E, Borght TV, Moreno E; Accuracy of DaTSCAN (123I-Ioflupane) SPECT in diagnosis of patients with clinically uncertain parkinsonism: 2-year follow-up of an open-label study. *Mov Disord* 2007;22(16):2346-51.

[20] Dethy S, Hambye AS. 1231-FP-CIT (DaTSCAN) scintigraphy in the differential diagnosis of movement disorders. *Rev Med Brux* 2008;29(4):238-47.

[21] Benamer HTS, Patterson J, Grosset DG. Accurate differentiation of parkinsonism and essential tremor using visual assessment of [123I]-FP-CIT SPECT imaging: the [123I]-FP-CIT SPECT study group. *Mov Disord* 2000;15:503-510.

[22] Marshall VL, Reininger CB, Marquardt M, et al. Parkinson's disease is overdiagnosed clinically at baseline in diagnostically uncertain cases: a 3-year European multicenter study with repeat [123I]-FP-CIT SPECT. *Mov Disord* 2009;24:500-508.

[23] Hauser RA, Grosset DG. [(123) I]FP-CIT (DaTscan) SPECT Brain Imaging in Patients with Suspected Parkinsonian Syndromes. *J Neuroimaging* 2012;22(3):225-230.

[24] Leinonen V, Menon LG, Carroll RS, Dello Iacono D, Grevet J, Jääskeläinen JE, Black PM. Cerebrospinal fluid biomarkers in idiopathic normal pressure hydrocephalus. *Int J Alzheimers Dis.* 2011;2011:312526. Epub 2011 Jun 1.

[25] Tarnaris A, Watkins LD, Kitchen ND. Biomarkers in chronic adult hydrocephalus. *Cerebrospinal Fluid Res* 2006;3:11.

[26] Kapaki EN, Paraskevas GP, Tzerakis NG, Sfagos C, Seretis A, Kararizou E, Vassilopoulos D. Cerebrospinal fluid tau, phospho-tau181 and beta-amyloid1-42 in idiopathic normal pressure hydrocephalus: a discrimination from Alzheimer's disease. *Eur J Neurol* 2007;14(2):168-173.

[27] Agren-Wilsson A, Lekman A, Sjöberg W, Rosengren L, Blennow K, Bergenheim AT, Malm J. CSF biomarkers in the evaluation of idiopathic normal pressure hydrocephalus. *Acta Neurol Scand* 2007;116(5):333-339.

[28] Tarnaris A, Toma AK, Kitchen ND, Watkins LD. Ongoing search for diagnostic biomarkers in idiopathic normal pressure hydrocephalus. *Biomark Med* 2009;3(6):787-805.

[29] Folstein MF, Folstein SE, McHugh PR. “Mini Mental State”: a practical method for grading the cognitive state of patients for the clinician. *J Psychiatr Res* 1975; 12:189-198.

[30] Dubois B, Slachevsky A, Litvan I, Pillon B. The FAB: a Frontal Assessment Battery at bedside. *Neurology* 2000 55, 1621-1626.

[31] Appollonio I, Leone M, Isella V, Piamarta F, Consoli T, Villa ML, Forapani E, Russo A, Nichelli P. et al. The Frontal Assessment Battery (FAB): normative values in an Italian population sample. *Neurol Sci* 2005 26, 108-116.

[32] Brazzelli M, Capitani E, Della Sala S, Spinnler H, Zuffi M. A neuropsychological instrument adding to the description of patients with suspected cortical dementia: the Milan overall dementia assessment *J Neurol, Neurosurg Psychiatry* 1994;57:1510-1517.

[33] Tinetti ME. Performance-oriented assessment of mobility problems in elderly patients. *J Am Geriatr Soc* 1986;34:119-126.

[34] Podsiadlo D, Richardson S. The timed ‘Up & Go’: A test of basic functional mobility for frail elderly persons. *J Am Geriatr Soc* 1991;39:142-148.

[35] Merello M, Nouzeilles MI, Arce GP, Leiguarda R. Accuracy of acute levodopa challenge for clinical prediction of sustained long-term levodopa response as a major criterion for idiopathic Parkinson’s Disease diagnosis. *Mov Disord.* 2002;17(4):795-798.

[36] Eide PK, Sorteberg W. Diagnostic intracranial pressure monitoring and surgical management in idiopathic normal pressure hydrocephalus: a 6-year review of 214 patients. *Neurosurgery* 2010;66:80-91.

[37] Klinge P, Hellstrom P, Tans J, et al. One-year outcome in the European multicentre study on iNPH. *Acta Neurol Scand* 2012;126:145-153.

[38] Farahmand D, Hilmarsson H, Hogfeldt M, et al. Perioperative risk factors for short term shunt revisions in adult hydrocephalus patients. *J Neurol Neurosurg Psychiatry* 2009;80:1248-1253.

[39] Wikkelsø C, Hellström P, Klinge PM, Tans JT; European iNPH Multicentre Study Group. The European iNPH Multicentre Study on the predictive values of resistance to CSF outflow and the CSF Tap Test in patients with idiopathic normal pressure hydrocephalus. *J Neurol Neurosurg Psychiatry*. 2013;84(5):562-568.

In: Parkinsonism
Editor: Cynthia Fisher
ISBN: 978-1-63483-865-8

Chapter 3

MAVRIDIS' ATROPHY

Ioannis N. Mavridis*
Department of Neurosurgery, 'K.A.T.-N.R.C.'
General Hospital of Attica, Athens, Greece

ABSTRACT

Parkinson's disease (PD), a common neurologic disorder of dopamine (DA) dysfunction, is characterized by motor, cognitive, psychiatric and autonomic symptoms. The nucleus accumbens (NA), a major part of the ventral striatum, belongs to the basal ganglia of the brain. It acts as a limbic-motor interface and plays an important role in motivation and emotional processes. It is the most important pleasure center of the human brain and is involved in some of the most disabling neuropsychiatric disorders, such as PD. More specifically, the NA is crucially involved in PD, not only in its pathogenesis and clinical manifestations but in the effects of several treatment efforts as well. Mavridis' atrophy (MA) is called the parkinsonism-related shrinkage of the human NA. The purpose of this chapter is to review the current knowledge regarding the role of MA in PD. MA was recently described as a novel research (neuroimaging) finding and there are subsequent important clinical studies confirming this finding. MA is part of the degeneration of the DAergic nigrostriatal system that occurs in PD and

* Correspondence: Ioannis N. Mavridis, M.D., Ph.D., Department of Neurosurgery, 'K.A.T.-N.R.C.' General Hospital of Attica, Nikis str. 2, Kifissia, 14561 Athens, Greece, Tel.: +306978327199, Fax: +302102833600, Email: pap-van@otenet.gr

this also explains the fact that MA precedes clinical phenotype. Thus, neuronal loss is probably the major cause of MA and, interestingly, degeneration of limbic areas is considered as a pathological consequence of MA. Functional NA changes also accompany MA. It has been shown that MA begins in early-stage PD patients and is correlated with psychiatric symptoms that occur in PD, mainly apathy and impulsive behavior. Moreover, MA is also associated with cognitive PD symptoms. Given that some motor and psychiatric symptoms may share a common pathophysiological process mediated by the NA, the clinical effects of MA are expected to include, apart from neuropsychiatric symptoms, motor symptoms as well; a hypothesis, however, that remains to be confirmed. MA, as an imaging finding, could be used as a risk factor for the expression and/or severity of specific symptoms, such as psychiatric manifestations, in PD patients. Further research is mandatory to enrich our knowledge and improve our understanding of the significance of the role of the MA phenomenon in PD. Future research efforts should focus on the underlying mechanisms of MA, its pathological features, as well as the clinical applications of this imaging finding.

Keywords: Dopamine, Mavridis' atrophy, neuropsychiatric symptoms, nucleus accumbens, Parkinson's disease

Introduction

Parkinson's disease (PD), a common neurologic disease, is an archetypal disorder of dopamine (DA) dysfunction characterized by motor, cognitive, behavioral and autonomic symptoms [1]. Beside the classically described motor manifestations, neuropsychiatric symptoms occur in the majority of patients and should be considered as an integral part of the disease [2, 3]. PD neuropsychiatric sequel includes dementia (subcortical or cortical) and cognitive impairment (including executive, visuospatial, attentional and memory dysfunctions), depression (common in early as well as in advanced PD [4]), dysthymia, anxiety disorders (including panic attacks), psychosis, apathy, sleep disorders (insomnia, parasomnias, somnolence, sleep attacks), sexual disorders and treatment-related psychiatric symptoms (ranging from vivid dreams and hallucinations to delusions, manic symptoms, hypersexuality, DA dysregulation syndrome and delirium) [3-9]. Furthermore, neuropsychiatric symptoms are important determinants of mortality, disease progression and patients' and caregivers' quality of life [3, 6-8].

PD has been associated with well-documented morphological changes in basal ganglia nuclei [10]. The striatum, the first relay of the basal ganglia system, is critically involved in motor functions and motivational processes. The dorsal striatum is central to the motor control and motor learning and the ventral striatum, especially the nucleus accumbens (NA) (Figure 1), is essential for motivation, the reward system and reinforcement by drugs. This system is dysfunctional in movement disorders such as PD and in psychiatric disorders [11]. Beside DAergic degeneration, with disease progression, non-DAergic nuclei, such as the locus coeruleus, the nucleus basalis of Meynert and the dorsal raphe, are affected [1].

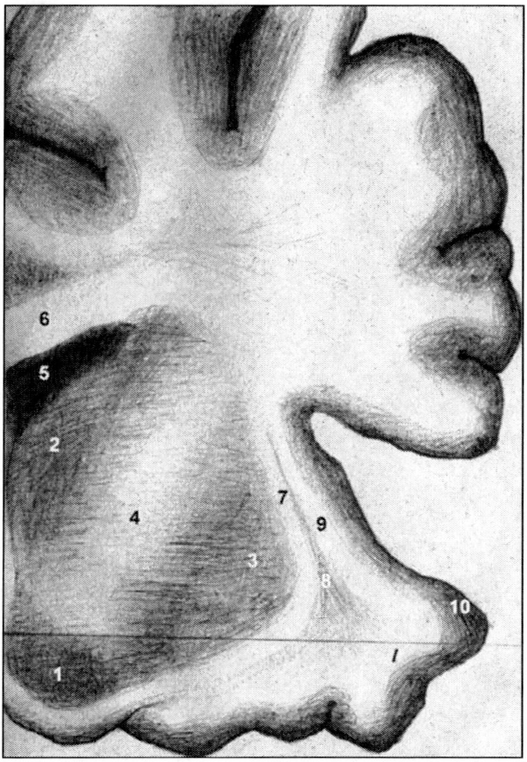

Figure 1. Anatomic location of the human NA within the frontal lobe (left cerebral hemisphere, coronal section 2 mm anterior to the anterior commissure). 1, NA; 2, head of the caudate nucleus; 3, putamen; 4, anterior limb of the internal capsule; 5, frontal horn of the lateral ventricle; 6, body of the corpus callosum; 7, external capsule; 8, claustrum; 9, extreme capsule; 10, insular cortex; *l*, intercommissural plane; NA, nucleus accumbens.

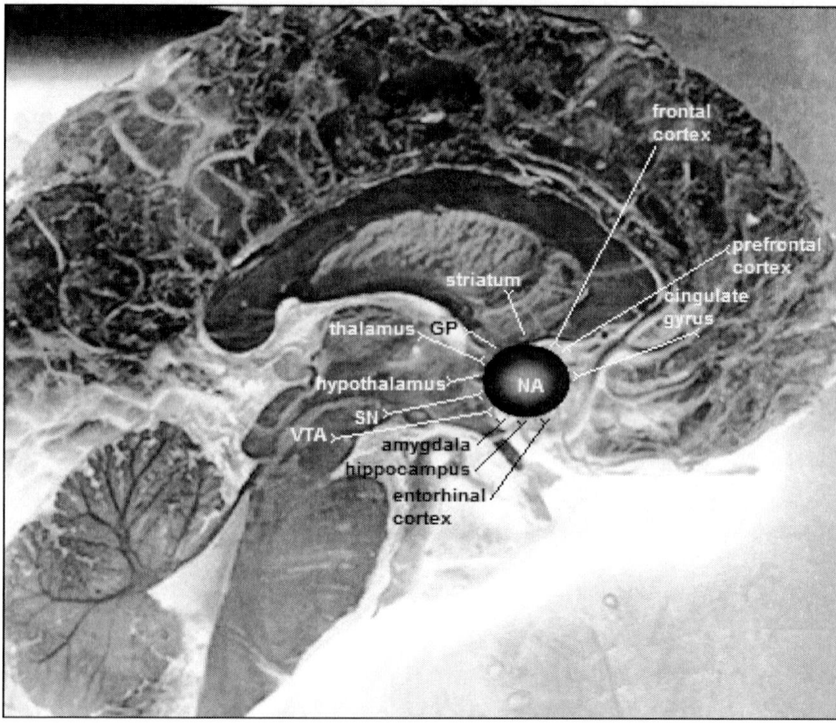

Figure 2. Summary of the connectivity between the NA and other cortical and subcortical structures (superimposed on the internal hemispheric surface). Synaptic terminals depict whether the shown connections are afferent, efferent or bidirectional. GP, globus pallidus; NA, nucleus accumbens; SN, substantia nigra; VTA, ventral tegmental area (modified from [12]).

The human NA, having DA as a principal neurotransmitter and dominating the reward system as a 'pleasure center', consists of two parts; a shell laterally and a core medialy. The first is mainly connected to the limbic and the second to the extrapyramidal motor system [12, 13]. Figure 2 summarizes the main cortical and subcortical afferent and efferent connections of the NA. Acting as a limbic-motor interface, the NA plays an important role in motivation and emotional processes, and is involved in some of the most common and disabling neuropsychiatric disorders, such as PD [12-17]. Table 1 summarizes the main neurologic and psychiatric conditions wherein the NA is involved [12]. The role of the NA neurotransmitters and neurons in PD has been established [18-21]. Specifically, this nucleus is crucially involved in PD, not only in its pathogenesis and clinical manifestations, but in the effects of several treatment efforts as well [14, 22]. Finally, it was recently found that the human NA suffers parkinsonism-related shrinkage, which is called Mavridis' atrophy (MA) [22-29].

Table 1. The main neurologic and psychiatric conditions wherein the NA is involved

Neurologic conditions	
-	Alzheimer's disease
-	Parkinson's disease
-	Epilepsy
-	Pain
-	Frontotemporal dementia
-	Tourette syndrome
-	Huntington's chorea
-	Narcolepsy
Psychiatric conditions	
-	Addiction (drugs, alcohol, smoking, gambling, etc.)
-	Depression
-	Anxiety disorders
-	Obsessive-compulsive disorder
-	Schizophrenia
-	Bipolar disorder
-	Attention-deficit / hyperactivity disorder
-	Posttraumatic stress disorder
-	Severe mood dysregulation
-	Apathy
-	Anorexia nervosa
-	Obesity
NA, nucleus accumbens	

Nowadays, almost two centuries after the publication of Dr. Parkinson's famous essay ("*An Essay on the Shaking Palsy*"), PD is considered as a thoroughly studied disease, with a lot of research efforts dealing with it, either from a clinical or from a basic-science point of view. But does this mean that we know PD well? We obviously do not and new research findings such as MA indicate that we have still a lot to learn about this disorder. The purpose of this chapter is to review the current knowledge regarding the role of MA in PD.

Nucleus Accumbens and Parkinson's Disease

Basic Science Data

Basic science studies have offered a lot in the improvement of our understanding of PD pathophysiology. PD models (produced with neurotoxins that selectively lesion DAergic neurons) are characterized by acute removal and gradual recovery of DA [30]. Slowly progressive loss of DA in ipsilateral NA following profound acute unilateral depletion of DA has been reported in the caudate-putamen of neonatal rats, with markedly increased metabolic turnover of DA in ipsilateral NA [30]. Severely decreased DA transporter binding in the ipsilateral caudate-putamen, NA and substantia nigra has been also reported in a rat model of PD [31]. Further, adenylyl cyclase supersensitivity has been observed in the NA of mice pretreated with twice-daily pramipexole and quinpirole, a finding possibly related to the exacerbation of gambling in PD that is provoked by antiparkinsonic agents acting as selective D2/D3 receptor agonists, notably pramipexole [32].

Data from neuropathological studies have indicated an association between the NA and PD. In Guam parkinsonism-dementia complex, for example, the large neurons in the neostriatum and NA degenerate while extremely severe (> 90%) loss of large neurons occurs in the NA. The latter may be linked to marked degeneration of limbic areas, ventral tegmental area (VTA) and nucleus dorsal raphe. The remaining large neurons and many of the medium-sized neurons in the NA are immunopositive for tau protein and contain various amounts of paired helical filaments admixed with straight tubules. Curly fibers and circularly arranged reactive astrocytes have been seen in the NA of many parkinsonism-dementia complex patients [33].

Clinical Data

Neuroimaging Findings

Imaging data regarding the NA role in PD are mainly provided by positron emission tomography (PET) studies of parkinsonic patients. Thus, increased 6-[(18)F]fluoro-l-DOPA utilization has been found in the bilateral medial NA in a group of patients with early, asymmetric PD. This finding suggests hyperfunction of catecholamine fibers innervating specifically the limbic striatum [34]. In contrast, another PET study in PD patients showed normal metabolic activity of the NA [35].

Interestingly, the level of DA transporter radiotracer binding in the NA and orbitofrontal cortex on the unaffected side, in early unilateral parkinsonism, is positively correlated with the conversion (from unilateral to bilateral parkinsonism) interval. This correlation indicates that the more severe a dysfunction in the mesocortical DAergic system (NA, caudate nucleus, orbitofrontal cortex) of the seemingly intact side, the more rapidly the parkinsonism proceeds to the intact side (bilateral parkinsonism). Moreover, the finding of bilateral reduction in the striatal radiotracer binding even in early stage (Hoehn and Yahr stage 1) PD patients confirms that molecular changes in the DAergic system precede clinical phenotype [36].

Furthermore, the specific (18)F-9-fluoropropyl-(+)-dihydrotetrabenzazine (a useful imaging marker to measure DAergic integrity) uptake ratios (in PET scans) of bilateral (in contrast to the unilateral nature of symptoms) caudate nucleus, putamen, substantia nigra and NA have been found to be significantly lower in PD patients at early stage of the disease with mild and unilateral motor symptoms. Consequently DAergic degeneration seems to take place in the premotor phase of PD [37].

Neuropsychiatric Manifestations

Neuropsychiatric symptoms that occur in PD such as depression, apathy, anxiety and anhedonia have a DAergic basis [38]. Involvement of the NA in such neuropsychiatric conditions has been reported [39-41]. Further, levodopa administered in a pulsatile manner may lead to the induction of synaptic plasticity within the DAergic systems. In the ventral mesolimbic system, this could lead to loss of behavioral flexibility, impulsive behavior and cognitive impairment [42].

Impulse control disorders and DA dysregulation syndrome in PD are motivation-based behaviors that involve repetitive occurrences of impulsive and uncontrolled activity [43]. Interestingly, DAergic replacement therapy in PD patients is among the most common causes of punding. Punding, drug-induced stereotypies, addiction and dyskinesias all share a common pathophysiological process. Punding may be related to plastic changes in the ventral and dorsal striatal structures, including the NA, and linked to psychomotor stimulation and reward mechanisms [44].

Based on data regarding psychiatric symptoms in PD patients subjected to chronic subthalamic nucleus (STN) deep brain stimulation (DBS), Haegelen et al. [45] proposed a new function scheme of the limbic system, establishing connections between limbic cortical structures and limbic part of the basal ganglia. This could be composed of a minor part based on the model of cortico-basal ganglia-thalamo-cortical loop and of a major part linking the STN with the mesolimbic DAergic pathway via the VTA and NA, and with limbic cortical structures. This scheme could explain limbic impairments after STN DBS by disruption of limbic information inside the STN and VTA [45].

Motor Manifestations

Despite the denial of the depressive state and the absence of obvious cognitive disorder, PD patients lack ambition and spend their time idly. However, although their motor function remains subliminal, such patients can carry out motor activities when the situation requires, but usually they do not have the drive to move [46]. The DAergic system of the dorsal striatal pathway projecting from the substantia nigra pars compacta to the dorsal part of the striatum (motor striatum) functions in the control of speed and dexterity of movement. On the other hand, the DAergic system, through the medial forebrain bundle projecting from the VTA to the NA, ventral striatum (limbic striatum) and cerebral cortex, is associated with hypokinesia and bradyphrenia [46].

The DA levels have been found relatively high in the NA of PD patients treated with levodopa, a finding possibly responsible for the occurrence of dyskinesias [47]. In contrast, the transient and reversible DA loss in the NA may contribute to the initial profound akinesia exhibited by common marmosets treated with 1-methyl-4-phenyl-1,2,3,6-tetrahydropyridine [48].

It is quite interesting the fact that endurance exercise has a beneficial effect on reactivity and movement behavior in PD patients following cued application of levodopa, probably due to an augmented synthesis and release of DA and other catecholamines in the prefrontal cortex, the NA and basal ganglia [49].

Furthermore, it has been found that PD patients do not present the normal pattern of greater activation of some brain areas including the left NA/caudate nucleus during motor timing [50].

Finally, in a PET study of PD patients who underwent STN DBS operations, the STN DBS-on condition during exercise (right-foot movement) significantly reduced the [(11)C]raclopride binding potential in the caudate nucleus and NA, but not in the putamen. The magnitude of DA release in the NA correlated negatively with the magnitude of motor load, indicating that STN DBS facilitated motor behavior more smoothly and at less expense to DAergic neurons in the region. The lack of DA release in the putamen and the significant DA release in the ventromedial striatum by STN DBS indicated DAergic activation occurring in the motivational circuit during action, suggesting a compensatory functional activation of the motor loop from the non-motor system [51].

Summary of the Nucleus Accumbens Role in Parkinson's Disease

It is clear that the NA is involved in several, not only psychiatric but also motor, symptoms occurring in PD patients, which fits better the functional profile of this nucleus (limbic-motor interface). Although the exact nature of this involvement is not fully understood, we know that the effects of the NA in the clinical expression of PD are associated with several pathological and pathophysiological changes. Table 2 summarizes the role of the NA in PD.

Table 2. Summary of the NA role in PD

❖ The NA is involved in psychiatric manifestations of PD.
❖ The NA is involved in motor symptoms occurring in PD patients.
❖ The NA effects in the clinical expression of PD are associated with pathological and pathophysiological changes.
❖ The exact nature of the NA involvement in PD is not fully understood.
NA, nucleus accumbens; PD, Parkinson's disease

Focus on Mavridis' Atrophy

Past: In Front of a New Finding

Discovery, Initial Hypotheses and Questions

As previously mentioned, there is robust data connecting molecular and/or cellular NA changes with the expression of PD. However, although atrophy of specific basal ganglia nuclei, such as the putamen [10], in PD is well established knowledge, such an observation regarding the NA was not reported in these patients until recently. Thus, NA atrophy in PD, nowadays called 'Mavridis' atrophy' [22-29], was discovered in 2010 (published in 2011) as an imaging finding [14]. It was, specifically, found that severe parkinsonism causes remarkable NA shrinkage (atrophy), namely 11.77% reduction in its relative size (on magnetic resonance images) [14] (Figure 3). These findings were the first to indicate in vivo that PD is associated with NA atrophy [52].

A combination of neuronal loss, neuronal shrinkage and reduction of synaptic terminals into the NA had been initially proposed as the potential cause of MA [14]. Two basic questions were raised with the discovery of MA [14, 16]:

1) Is this phenomenon also observed in patients with early PD?
2) Is this atrophy correlated with the neuropsychiatric symptoms that occur in PD?

It had been then proposed that MA could be related to DAergic neuropsychiatric symptoms (mediated by a malfunctioning NA) that occur in PD, as well as to its comorbidity with other psychiatric conditions such as depression [14]. A potential role (even as a predictive factor) in PD comorbidity with psychiatric conditions had been also suggested for MA [14].

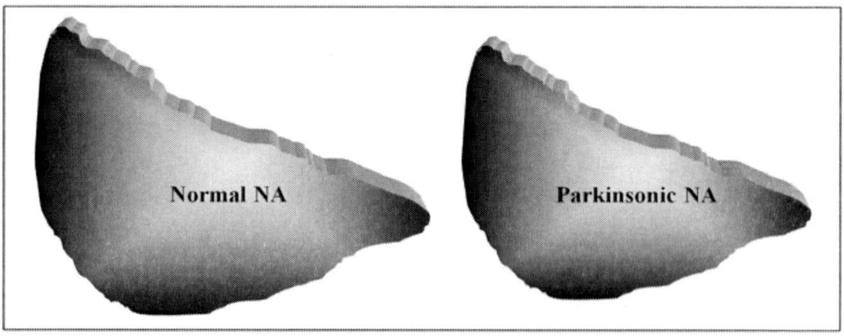

Figure 3. Schematic representation of the difference between the size of a normal and a parkinsonic (atrophic) NA, which is 11.77% smaller. NA: nucleus accumbens.

Later Suggestions

Neuronal loss due to DAergic degeneration was later supported as the major cause of MA. Functional NA changes such as decreased DA, nuclear dysfunction (decreased activation) and changes in its synaptic plasticity were suggested to accompany MA [22]. Degeneration of limbic areas could be easily considered as a pathological consequence of MA and neuropsychiatric (mainly due to limbic dysfunction) and motor symptoms (mainly negative) were also proposed as its clinical effects [22]. Thus, NA might be associated with the neuropsychiatric non-motor symptoms that are present in the disease, like depression and anxiety [52]. Regarding the inclusion of motor symptoms in the clinical consequences of MA, this seems to be a rational hypothesis given the aforementioned NA role in PD [22].

Furthermore, the MA, as an imaging finding, has been suggested as a predictive factor for the development of psychiatric manifestations such as depression (and probably of other symptoms too) that occur in PD [22]. Finally, given that DAergic degeneration takes place in the premotor phase [37] of PD and that molecular changes in the DAergic system precede clinical phenotype of PD [36], a MA onset in early PD was supported [22]. Despite all the above mentioned hypotheses, a definite conclusion could not be made based on the available research data at the time.

Recent Clinical Studies and the First Answers

Recently, clinical research has offered new insight in the field. At first, two studies by O'Callaghan et al. [53, 54], published in 2013, confirmed the finding of MA. And it was the recent study by Lee et al. (2014) [55] which provided a definite answer to the first of the initial questions that accompanied the MA discovery. According to their results, untreated, early stage PD patients without dementia had significant reductions in adjusted NA volumes [55]. Thus they not only confirmed the MA phenomenon but also proved that it occurs in early stages of the disease.

Neuropsychiatric Symptoms

Regarding the second initially arisen question, three recent studies provided affirmative answers [53, 56, 57]. O'Callaghan et al. [53], in 2013, provided evidence that disinhibition (inhibitory dysfunction is a key feature of impulsive behavior) in PD is related to fronto-striatal gray matter atrophy. They specifically found that, in PD patients, right NA atrophy was associated with response disinhibition. They supported the hypothesis that fronto-striatal structural abnormalities contribute to impulsive behaviors in these patients [53].

According to the results of Lee et al. (2014) [57], PD patients with medication-related impulse control disorders showed tendency to lower binding potentials (in PET scans) at the left NA compared with those free of impulse control disorders. The impulse control disorders subjects also showed reduced uptakes at both ventral striatal regions. The authors concluded that a great gap in extrastriatal versus striatal DAergic fiber degeneration is an intrinsic condition predisposing to impulse control disorders in PD [57]. We should remember here that DAergic degeneration was suggested as the major cause of MA [22].

Finally, Carriere et al. (2014) [56] found that DA-refractory apathy in PD was associated with atrophy of the left NA. They also found a positive correlation between the severity of apathy and atrophy of the left NA, as well as greater atrophy in the bilateral NA in apathetic patients than in controls [56]. So, their study confirmed the MA finding and proved its correlation with a specific psychiatric symptom of PD, namely apathy. The lateralization of findings in all these three studies (regarding psychiatric PD symptoms) is a quite interesting observation, which requires further research in order to clarify its potential significance.

Cognitive Symptoms

Interestingly, two recent studies suggested that MA is associated with cognitive PD symptoms as well [54, 58]. O'Callaghan et al. (2013) [54] found that learning rates were reduced in non-demented PD patients relative to controls and that this learning impairment was directly related to gray matter loss in discrete fronto-striatal regions including the NA.

Additionally, according to the results of Hanganu et al. (2014) [58], a significant decrease in the volume of the NA was observed specifically in patients with PD with mild cognitive impairment. These results indicate that the early presence of mild cognitive impairment in patients with PD is associated with a significant diminishment of limbic subcortical structures. This specific pattern of brain degradation associated with the early presence of mild cognitive impairment might serve as a marker of development toward dementia [58].

Present: Where We Are Now

Thanks to the above mentioned recent clinical research data, we are nowadays able to have at least some insight in the formerly unknown MA role in PD and some definite answers as well. We currently know that MA, a confirmed by subsequent studies finding, is part of the degeneration of the DAergic nigrostriatal system that occurs in PD and this also explains the fact that MA precedes clinical phenotype [59]. So, MA begins in early-stage PD patients [55] and is correlated with neuropsychiatric symptoms that occur in PD, including apathy, impulsive behavior and disinhibition [53, 56, 57]. It is also associated with cognitive PD symptoms such as learning and cognitive impairment [54, 58]. Table 3 summarizes the current knowledge regarding the role of the MA phenomenon in PD.

Table 3. What we currently know about the MA role in PD

❖	MA is a new research finding that has been confirmed by recent studies.
❖	MA is part of the degeneration of the DAergic nigrostriatal system that occurs in PD.
❖	MA begins in early-stage PD patients.
❖	MA is correlated with neuropsychiatric symptoms that occur in PD (apathy, impulsive behavior, disinhibition).
❖	MA is associated with cognitive PD symptoms (learning impairment, cognitive impairment).
❖	We have still a lot to learn about the role of MA (and its value as an imaging finding) in PD.

NA, nucleus accumbens; PD, Parkinson's disease

Future: Remaining Questions, Challenges and Clinical Applications

In spite of having the first answers to some vital questions regarding MA, we are currently seeing just the 'peak' of the largely 'unexplored iceberg' called 'MA' [26]. Some crucial questions that still remain to be answered include [26, 27, 59]:

1) Does the human NA follow the same (as other basal ganglia nuclei) pattern of DAergic degeneration?
2) What kind of microscopic pathological changes do characterize this atrophy?
3) Do all parkinsonics suffer MA?
4) Is this phenomenon also associated with motor PD symptoms?

It would be therefore essential to have a post-mortem pathological study focused on the NA of parkinsonic individuals [59], as well as clinical studies focusing on the potential association between the NA morphology and motor manifestations of PD.

Finally, it is time to evaluate MA (as an imaging finding) as a risk factor for the expression and/or severity of specific PD symptoms, emphasizing on those we already know that are related to MA (namely psychiatric and cognitive symptoms), and even as a prognostic factor for the severity of the disease [26, 59]. It remains to be tested whether the severity of MA affects the severity of specific psychiatric symptoms (apathy, compulsive behavior) of parkinsonic individuals and whether the presence of MA is related with the expression and/or severity of motor PD symptoms. Such clinical studies, that could provide answers to these vital questions, could be easily preformed given the high frequency of PD in modern populations. In this direction, future research efforts are mandatory to enrich our knowledge of MA [27], namely its underlying mechanisms, its pathological features and clinical consequences [59], as well as its potential prognostic value in PD patients.

Conclusion

PD is a common neurologic disorder of DA dysfunction characterized by motor, cognitive, behavioral and autonomic symptoms, while neuropsychiatric symptoms are an integral part of the disease. PD is associated with well-documented morphological changes in basal ganglia nuclei, including the NA. The latter, having DA as a principal neurotransmitter and dominating the reward system, is connected to the limbic and extrapyramidal motor system. Acting as a limbic-motor interface, the NA plays an important role in motivation and emotional processes, and is involved in some of the most common and disabling neuropsychiatric disorders, such as PD. This nucleus is crucially involved in PD, not only in its pathogenesis and clinical manifestations, but also in the effects of several treatment efforts. It is clear that the NA is involved in several not only psychiatric but also motor symptoms occurring in PD patients, which fits better the functional profile of this nucleus. Although the exact nature of this involvement is not fully understood, we know that the effects of the NA in the clinical expression of PD are associated with several pathological and pathophysiological changes.

The recent discovery of MA provided the pathological explanation of the NA role in PD and set this role into a different perspective. MA as a new research finding brought several vital questions necessitating answers, as well as several hypotheses about the significance and role of this phenomenon. Thanks to very recent clinical studies, this finding has been confirmed and we have the first answers. Thus, we currently know that MA is part of the degeneration of the DAergic nigrostriatal system that occurs in PD and this also explains the fact that MA precedes clinical phenotype. So, MA begins in early-stage PD patients and is correlated with neuropsychiatric symptoms that occur in PD, including apathy, impulsive behavior and disinhibition. It is also associated with cognitive PD symptoms such as learning and cognitive impairment. Further research is necessary for the improvement of our understanding of the MA in PD patients and to explore its potential usefulness as a risk factor for the expression and/or severity of specific PD symptoms and even as a prognostic factor for the severity of the disease. Future research efforts are expected to enrich our knowledge of the underlying mechanisms, pathological features and clinical consequences of MA.

REFERENCES

[1] Voon V, Fernagut PO, Wickens J, Baunez C, Rodriguez M, Pavon N, Juncos JL, Obeso JA, Bezard E. Chronic dopaminergic stimulation in Parkinson's disease: from dyskinesias to impulse control disorders. *Lancet Neurol.* 2009;8:1140-9.

[2] Arsland D, Larsen JP. [Emotional and cognitive disorders in Parkinson disease]. *Tidsskr. Nor. Laegeforen.* 1998;118(25):3959-63. Norwegian.

[3] Aarsland D, Pedersen KF, Ehrt U, Bronnick K, Gjerstad MD, Larsen JP. [Neuropsychiatric and cognitive symptoms in Parkinson disease]. *Tidsskr. Nor. Laegeforen.* 2008;128(18):2072-6. Norwegian.

[4] Schrag A. Psychiatric aspects of Parkinson's disease--an update. *J. Neurol.* 2004;251(7):795-804.

[5] Mindham RH. Psychiatric symptoms in Parkinsonism. *J. Neurol. Neurosurg. Psychiatry* 1970;33(2):188-91.

[6] Aarsland D, Karlsen K. Neuropsychiatric aspects of Parkinson's disease. *Curr. Psychiatry Rep.* 1999;1(1):61-8.

[7] Lauterbach EC. The neuropsychiatry of Parkinson's disease and related disorders. *Psychiatr. Clin. North Am.* 2004;27(4):801-25.

[8] Lauterbach EC. The neuropsychiatry of Parkinson's disease. *Minerva Med.* 2005;96(3):155-73.

[9] Kalaitzakis ME, Graeber MB, Gentleman SM, Pearce RK. Striatal beta-amyloid deposition in Parkinson disease with dementia. *J. Neuropathol. Exp. Neurol.* 2008;67(2):155-61.

[10] Geng DY, Li YX, Zee CS. Magnetic resonance imagingbased volumetric analysis of basal ganglia nuclei and substantia nigra in patients with Parkinson's disease. *Neurosurgery* 2006;58(2):256-62.

[11] Schiffmann SN. [Changes in neural networks by conditional transgenic approach: a key to our comprehension of neuro-psychiatric disorders in the basal ganglia system]. *Bull. Mem. Acad. R. Med. Belg.* 2009;164(7-9):171-8; discussion 178-80. French.

[12] Mavridis IN. [Stereotactic neurosurgical anatomy of the nucleus accumbens]. PhD Thesis, National and Kapodistrian University of

Athens (School of Medicine), Athens, Greece, 2012, doi: 10.12681/eadd/27603. Greek.

[13] Mavridis IN. Music and the nucleus accumbens. *Surg. Radiol. Anat.* 2015;37(2):121-5.

[14] Mavridis I, Boviatsis E, Anagnostopoulou S. The human nucleus accumbens suffers parkinsonism-related shrinkage: a novel finding. *Surg. Radiol. Anat.* 2011;33(7):595-9.

[15] Mavridis I. [The role of the nucleus accumbens in neurological disorders]. *Neurologia-gr* 2012;21(6):6-11. Greek.

[16] Mavridis I, Boviatsis E, Anagnostopoulou S. Parkinsonism-related shrinkage of the human nucleus accumbens: a novel finding. In: 14th European Congress of Neurosurgery, October 9-14, 2011, Rome, Italy-*Abstracts CD*. The European Association of Neurosurgical Societies, 2011; Oral presentations, Parallel session: Functional Neurosurgery, No 181.

[17] Mavridis I, Boviatsis E, Anagnostopoulou S. Anatomy of the human nucleus accumbens: a combined morphometric study. *Surg. Radiol. Anat.* 2011;33(5):405-14.

[18] Elsworth JD, Taylor JR, Sladek JR Jr, Collier TJ, Redmond DE Jr, Roth RH. Striatal dopaminergic correlates of stable parkinsonism and degree of recovery in old-world primates one year after MPTP treatment. *Neuroscience* 2000;95(2):399-408.

[19] Ikemoto K. Human striatal D-neurons and their significance. *Nihon Shinkei Seishin Yakurigaku Zasshi* 2002;22(4):131-5.

[20] Tong J, Hornykiewicz O, Kish SJ. Inverse relationship between brain noradrenaline level and dopamine loss in Parkinson disease. A possible neuroprotective role for noradrenaline. *Arch. Neurol.* 2006;63(12):1724-8.

[21] Cools R, Lewis SJG, Clark L, Barker RA, Robbins TW. L-dopa disrupts activity in the nucleus accumbens during reversal learning in Parkinson's disease. *Neuropsychopharmacology* 2007;32(1):180-9.

[22] Mavridis IN. Nucleus accumbens and Parkinson's disease: exploring the role of Mavridis' atrophy. *OA Case Rep.* 2014;3(4):35.

[23] Mavridis IN. Stereotactic neurosurgical anatomy of the nucleus accumbens: four-year outcomes. *Surg. Radiol. Anat.* 2013;35(7):637-8.

[24] Mavridis IN. Anatomizing the "King of Neurosciences." *World J. Neurol.* 2013;3(2):4-6.

[25] Mavridis IN. Mavridis' atrophy begins in early stage Parkinson's disease. *Parkinsonism Relat. Disord.* 2014;20(11):1323.

[26] Mavridis IN. Mavridis' atrophy in Parkinson's disease: "The peak of the iceberg." *J. Transl. Intern. Med.* 2014;2(3):124-6.

[27] Mavridis IN. Nucleus accumbens and Parkinson's disease: The role of Mavridis' atrophy. In: World Psychiatric Association Thematic Conference on Intersectional Collaboration & 5th European Congress of the International Neuropsychiatric Association & 2nd Interdisciplinary Congress "Psychiatry and Related Sciences," October 30-November 1, 2014, Athens, Greece-*Book of Abstracts*. World Psychiatric Association & International Neuropsychiatric Association & Hellenic Society for the Advancement of Psychiatry and Related Sciences, 2014; Free Communications, FC5.1.

[28] Mavridis IN. Is nucleus accumbens atrophy correlated with cognitive symptoms of Parkinson's disease? *Brain* 2015;138(Pt 1):e319.

[29] Mavridis IN. We know now: Mavridis' atrophy is associated with cognitive impairment in Parkinson's disease. *AJNR Am. J. Neuroradiol.* 2015;36(5):E38.

[30] Teicher MH, Andersen SL, Campbell A, Gelbard HA, Baldessarini RJ. Progressive accumbens degeneration after neonatal striatal 6-hydroxydopamine in rats. *Neurosci. Lett.* 1998;247(2-3):99-102.

[31] Casteels C, Lauwers E, Bormans G, Baekelandt V, Van Laere K. Metabolic-dopaminergic mapping of the 6-hydroxydopamine rat model for Parkinson's disease. *Eur. J. Nucl. Med. Mol. Imaging* 2008;35(1):124-34.

[32] Aloisi G, Silvano E, Rossi M, Millan MJ, Maggio R. Differential induction of adenylyl cyclase supersensitivity by antiparkinson drugs acting as agonists at dopamine D1/D2/D3 receptors vs D2/D3 receptors only: parallel observations from co-transfected human and native cerebral receptors. *Neuropharmacology* 2011;60(2-3):439-45.

[33] Oyanagi K, Makifuchi T, Ohtoh T, Chen KM, Gajdusek DC, Chase TN, Ikuta F. The neostriatum and nucleus accumbens in parkinsonism-dementia complex of Guam: a pathological comparison with Alzheimer's disease and progressive supranuclear palsy. *Acta Neuropathol.* 1994;88(2):122-8.

[34] Kumakura Y, Danielsen EH, Gjedde A, Vernaleken I, Buchholz HG, Heinz A, Gründer G, Bartenstein P, Cumming P. Elevated [(18)F]FDOPA utilization in the periaqueductal gray and medial nucleus accumbens of patients with early Parkinson's disease. *Neuroimage* 2010;49(4):2933-9.

[35] Eggers C, Hilker R, Burghaus L, Schumacher B, Heiss WD. High resolution positron emission tomography demonstrates basal ganglia dysfunction in early Parkinson's disease. *J. Neurol. Sci.* 2009;276(1-2):27-30.

[36] Yagi S, Yoshikawa E, Futatsubashi M, Yokokura M, Yoshihara Y, Torizuka T, Ouchi Y. Progression from unilateral to bilateral parkinsonism in early Parkinson disease: implication of mesocortical dopamine dysfunction by PET. *J. Nucl Med.* 2010;51(8):1250-7.

[37] Lin SC, Lin KJ, Hsiao IT, Hsieh CJ, Lin WY, Lu CS, Wey SP, Yen TC, Kung MP, Weng YH. In vivo detection of monoaminergic degeneration in early Parkinson disease by (18)F-9-fluoropropyl-(+)-dihydrotetrabenzazine PET. *J. Nucl. Med.* 2014;55(1):73-9.

[38] Chaudhuri KR, Schapira AHV. Non-motor symptoms of Parkinson's disease: dopaminergic pathophysiology and treatment. *Lancet Neurol.* 2009;8(5):464-74.

[39] Sturm V, Lenartz D, Koulousakis A, Treuer H, Herholz K, Klein JC, Klosterkötter J. The nucleus accumbens: a target for deep brain stimulation in obsessive-compulsive and anxiety disorders. *J. Chem. Neuroanat.* 2003;26(4):293-9.

[40] Paul RH, Brickman AM, Navia B, Hinkin C, Malloy PF, Jefferson AL, Cohen RA, Tate DF, Flanigan TP. Apathy is associated with volume of the nucleus accumbens in patients infected with HIV. *J. Neuropsychiatry Clin. Neurosci.* 2005;17(2):167-71.

[41] Schlaepfer TE, Cohen MX, Frick C, Kosel M, Brodesser D, Axmacher N, Joe AY, Kreft M, Lenartz D, Sturm V. Deep brain stimulation to reward circuitry alleviates anhedonia in refractory major depression. *Neuropsychopharmacology* 2008;33(2):368-77.

[42] Grace AA. Physiology of the normal and dopamine-depleted basal ganglia: insights into levodopa pharmacotherapy. *Mov. Disord.* 2008;23 Suppl 3:S560-9.

[43] Okai D, Samuel M, Askey-Jones S, David AS, Brown RG. Impulse control disorders and dopamine dysregulation in Parkinson's disease: a broader conceptual framework. *Eur. J. Neurol.* 2011;18(12):1379-83.

[44] Fasano A, Petrovic I. Insights into pathophysiology of punding reveal possible treatment strategies. *Mol. Psychiatry* 2010;15(6):560-73.

[45] Haegelen C, Rouaud T, Darnault P, Morandi X. The subthalamic nucleus is a key-structure of limbic basal ganglia functions. *Med. Hypotheses* 2009;72(4):421-6.

[46] Yokochi M. [Mesolimbic and mesocortical pathways in Parkinson disease]. *Brain Nerve* 2007;59(9):943-51. Japanese.

[47] Goldstein M, Lieberman A, Pearson J. Relatively high levels of dopamine in nucleus accumbens of levodopa treated patients with Parkinson's disease. *J. Neural Transm.* 1982;54(1-2):129-34.

[48] Rose S, Nomoto M, Jenner P, Marsden CD. Transient depletion of nucleus accumbens dopamine content may contribute to initial akinesia induced by MPTP in common marmosets. *Biochem. Pharmacol.* 1989;38(21):3677-81.

[49] Müller T, Muhlack S. Effect of exercise on reactivity and motor behaviour in patients with Parkinson's disease. *J. Neurol. Neurosurg. Psychiatry* 2010;81(7):747-53.

[50] Jahanshahi M, Jones CR, Zijlmans J, Katzenschlager R, Lee L, Quinn N, Frith CD, Lees AJ. Dopaminergic modulation of striato-frontal connectivity during motor timing in Parkinson's disease. *Brain* 2010;133(Pt 3):727-45.

[51] Nozaki T, Sugiyama K, Yagi S, Yoshikawa E, Kanno T, Asakawa T, Ito T, Terada T, Namba H, Ouchi Y. Effect of subthalamic nucleus stimulation during exercise on the mesolimbocortical dopaminergic region in Parkinson's disease: a positron emission tomography study. *J. Cereb. Blood Flow Metab.* 2013;33(3):415-21.

[52] Monchi O, Hanganu A. Reply: is nucleus accumbens atrophy correlated with cognitive symptoms of Parkinson's disease? *Brain* 2015;138(Pt 1):e320.

[53] O'Callaghan C, Naismith SL, Hodges JR, Lewis SJ, Hornberger M. Fronto-striatal atrophy correlates of inhibitory dysfunction in Parkinson's disease versus behavioural variant frontotemporal dementia. *Cortex* 2013;49(7):1833-43.

[54] O'Callaghan C, Moustafa AA, de Wit S, Shine JM, Robbins TW, Lewis SJ, Hornberger M. Fronto-striatal gray matter contributions to discrimination learning in Parkinson's disease. *Front. Comput. Neurosci.* 2013;7:180.

[55] Lee HM, Kwon KY, Kim MJ, Jang JW, Suh SI, Koh SB, Kim JH. Subcortical grey matter changes in untreated, early stage Parkinson's disease without dementia. *Parkinsonism Relat. Disord.* 2014;20(6):622-6.

[56] Carriere N, Besson P, Dujardin K, Duhamel A, Defebvre L, Delmaire C, Devos D. Apathy in Parkinson's disease is associated with nucleus

accumbens atrophy: A magnetic resonance imaging shape analysis. *Mov. Disord.* 2014;29(7):897-903.

[57] Lee JY, Seo SH, Kim YK, Yoo HB, Kim YE, Song IC, Lee JS, Jeon BS. Extrastriatal dopaminergic changes in Parkinson's disease patients with impulse control disorders. *J. Neurol. Neurosurg. Psychiatry* 2014;85(1):23-30.

[58] Hanganu A, Bedetti C, Degroot C, Mejia-Constain B, Lafontaine AL, Soland V, Chouinard S, Bruneau MA, Mellah S, Belleville S, Monchi O. Mild cognitive impairment is linked with faster rate of cortical thinning in patients with Parkinson's disease longitudinally. *Brain* 2014;137(Pt 4):1120-9.

[59] Mavridis IN, Pyrgelis ES. Mavridis' atrophy in Parkinson's disease-five years later: future perspectives. *World J. Neurol.* 2015;5(1):1-4.

Peer review was arranged by Dr. Maria Meliou, MD

BIBLIOGRAPHY

A guide to the extrapyramidal side-effects of antipsychotic drugs LCCN: 2013039676 Personal name: Owens, D. G. Cunningham (David Griffith Cunningham), 1949- author. Main title: A guide to the extrapyramidal side-effects of antipsychotic drugs / D. G. Cunningham-Owens, Professor of Clinical Psychiatry, University of Edinburgh, Division of Psychiatry, Royal Edinburgh Hospital, Edinburgh, UK. Edition: Second edition. Published/Produced: Cambridge; New York: Cambridge University Press, [2014] ©2014 Description: viii, 377 pages: illustrations; 26 cm ISBN: 9781107022867 (hardback) 110702286X (hardback) LC classification: RM333.5 .O94 2014 Summary: "It is often implied that antipsychotic-induced extrapyramidal side-effects are irrelevant to modern psychiatric therapeutics, rendered historic by newer, better treatments. This myth arises from limited awareness of the depth and breadth of neurological disruption antipsychotics can mediate. This volume discusses the extensive clinical boundaries of acute dystonias, drug-induced parkinsonism, akathisia and tardive dyskinesia, providing demographic and epidemiological context while illustrating how prescribing choices impact powerfully on their development. This new edition has been thoroughly updated and rewritten to include recent data, expanded references and a new chapter on the concept of 'atypical' antipsychotics. Written in a light, engaging style, liberally illustrated with clinical examples, it also invites readers to consider ongoing controversies - subjective drug effects, the relationship between 'akathisia' and restless legs, the status of the concept of 'atypicality', and so on. Informative reading for trainees as well as established practitioners in the fields of psychiatry, neurology, primary care and geriatrics"--Provided by publisher. Contents: Machine generated contents note: Preface; Part 1. Setting the Scene: 1. The origins of psychopharma; 2. Some preliminaries; Part 2. The Syndromes: 3. Acute dystonias; 4. Parkinsonism; 5. Akathisia; 6. Tardive dyskinesia; Part 3. Particular Issues: 7. Tardive and chronic dystonia; 8. Special populations; Part 4. Assessment: 9. The clinical examination; 10. An overview of some standardised recording instruments; Part 5. Matters Arising: 11. Involuntary movements and schizophrenia: a limitation to the concept of tardive dyskinesia?; 12. And finally ... the salutary tale of 'atypicality'; References; Index. Subjects: Basal Ganglia Diseases--chemically induced. Antipsychotic Agents--adverse effects. Extrapyramidal Tracts--drug effects. Neurotoxicity Syndromes. Notes: Includes bibliographical references (pages 320-370) and index.

A practical approach to movement disorders: diagnosis and management LCCN: 2014013970 Personal name: Fernandez, Hubert H., author. Main title: A practical approach to movement disorders: diagnosis and management / editors, Hubert H. Fernandez, Andre G. Machado, Mayur Pandya. Edition: Second edition. Published/Produced: New York, NY: Demos Medical Publishing, LLC, [2015] Description: xiv, 401 pages; 21 cm ISBN: 9781620700341 (print: alk. paper) LC classification: RC376.5 .P73 2015 Related names: Machado, Andre (Neurosurgeon), author. Pandya, Mayur, author. Contents: The body language of movement disorders -- Tremors -- Parkinsonism -- Parkinson's disease -- Dystonia -- Chorea -- Myoclonus -- Ataxia -- Tics -- Sleep-related movements -- The psychiatric assessment -- Psychiatric issues in Parkinson's disease -- Psychiatric issues in Huntington's disease -- Psychiatric issues in Tourette's syndrome -- Approach to conversion disorders -- Surgical approach to movement disorders -- Physical and occupational therapy -- Speech and swallowing therapy -- Nutritional considerations. Subjects: Movement Disorders--

Handbooks. Notes: Preceded by A practical approach to movement disorders / Hubert H. Fernandez ... [et al.]. c2007. Includes bibliographical references and index.

Clinical neuropsychology and cognitive neurology of Parkinson's disease and other movement disorders LCCN: 2014012805 Main title: Clinical neuropsychology and cognitive neurology of Parkinson's disease and other movement disorders / edited by Alexander I. Tröster. Published/Produced: Oxford; New York: Oxford University Press, [2015] ©2015 Description: xii, 546 pages: illustrations; 25 cm ISBN: 9780199812370 0199812373 LC classification: RC382 .C576 2015 Related names: Tröster, Alexander I., editor. Contents: Basal ganglia circuits: structure, function and dysfunction / Thomas Wichmann and Mahlon R. DeLong -- Neurocognitive screening and assessment in Parkinsonism / Jaime Kulisevsky and Javier Pagonabarraga -- A general approach to clinical neuropsychological assessment of movement disorders / Michele K. York and Adriana M. Strutt -- Movement disorders and their impact on quality of life / Delia Lorenz and Günther Deuschl -- Neuropathology, biomarkers, and cognition in Parkinson's disease / Eiron Cudaback, Brenna A. Cholerton, Kathleen S. Montine, and Thomas J. Montine -- Structural and functional neuroimaging of cognition and emotion in Parkinson's disease / Carme Junque -- Genetics and cognition in Parkinson's disease / Madeleine E. Sharp and Roy N. Alcalay -- Earliest cognitive changes and mild cognitive impairment in Parkinson's disease / Ben Schmand and Alexander I. Tröster -- Dementia in Parkinson's disease / Arvid Rongve, Eirik Auning, Astrid Haram, and Dag Aarsland -- Depression and anxiety in Parkinson's disease / Laura Marsh and Roseanne D. Dobkin -- Impulse control disorders, apathy, and psychosis in Parkinson's disease / Daniel Weintraub and Jennifer G. Goldman -- Effects of deep brain stimulation in movement disorders on cognition and behavior / Julie A. Fields -- Huntington's disease / Arshia Saddredin and Ioan Stroescu -- Corticobasal degeneration / Melissa Armstrong and Irene Litvan -- Multiple system atrophy / Kathy Dujardin and Luc Defebvre -- Progressive supranuclear palsy / Barbara Borroni and Alessandro Padovani

-- Neuropsychological and neuropsychiatric features of dystonia and the impact of medical and surgical treatment / Mariam Torkamani and Marjan Jahanshahi -- Essential tremor / Kelly E. Lyons and Alexander I. Tröster. Subjects: Parkinson's disease--Complications. Cognition disorders--Etiology. Movement disorders--Complications. Parkinson's disease--Psychological aspects. Movement disorders $x Psychological aspects. Parkinson Disease--complications. Cognition Disorders--etiology. Mental Disorders--etiology. Movement Disorders--complications. Neurobehavioral Manifestations. Parkinson Disease--psychology. Notes: Includes bibliographical references and index.

Hallucinations LCCN: 2012002877 Personal name: Sacks, Oliver W. Main title: Hallucinations / Oliver Sacks. Edition: 1st American ed. Published/Created: New York: Alfred A. Knopf, 2012. Description: xiv, 326 p.; 22 cm. Links: Contributor biographical information http://www.loc.gov/catdir/enhancements/fy1304/2012002877-b.html Publisher description http://www.loc.gov/catdir/enhancements/fy1304/2012002877-d.html Sample text http://www.loc.gov/catdir/enhancements/fy1304/2012002877-s.html ISBN: 9780307957245 0307957241 LC classification: RC553.H3 S23 2012 Summary: This book is an investigation into the types, physiological sources, and cultural resonances of hallucinations traces everything from the disorientations of sleep and intoxication to the manifestations of injury and illness. Have you ever seen something that was not really there? Heard someone call your name in an empty house? Sensed someone following you and turned around to find nothing? Hallucinations don't belong wholly to the insane. Much more commonly, they are linked to sensory deprivation, intoxication, illness, or injury. People with migraines may see shimmering arcs of light or tiny, Lilliputian figures of animals and people. People with failing eyesight, paradoxically, may become immersed in a hallucinatory visual world. Hallucinations can be brought on by a simple fever or even the act of waking or falling asleep, when people have visions ranging from luminous blobs of color to beautifully detailed faces or terrifying ogres. Those who are bereaved may receive comforting "visits" from the departed. In some conditions, hallucinations can lead to religious epiphanies or even the feeling of leaving one's own body. Humans have always sought such life-changing visions, and for thousands of years have used hallucinogenic compounds to achieve them. As a young doctor in California in the 1960s, the author had both a personal and a professional interest in psychedelics. These, along with his early migraine experiences, launched a lifelong investigation into the varieties of hallucinatory experience. Here, he weaves together stories of his patients and of his own mind-altering experiences to illuminate what hallucinations tell us about the organization and structure of our brains, how they have influenced every culture's folklore and art, and why the potential for hallucination is present in us all, a vital part of the human condition.-- Source other than Library of Congress. Contents: Silent multitudes: Charles Bonnet Syndrome -- The prisoner's cinema: sensory deprivation -- A few nanograms of wine: hallucinatory smells -- Hearing things -- The illusions of Parkinsonism -- Altered states -- Patterns: visual migraines -- The "sacred" disease -- Bisected: hallucinations in the half-field -- Delirious -- On the threshold of sleep -- Narcolepsy and night hags -- The haunted mind -- Doppelgängers: hallucinating oneself -- Phantoms, shadows, and sensory ghosts. Subjects: Hallucinations and illusions. Cognition disorders. Perceptual disorders. Hallucinations. Perceptual Disorders. Notes: Includes bibliographical references (p. 297-309) and index.

Handbook of Parkinson's disease LCCN: 2013444071 Main title: Handbook of Parkinson's disease / edited by Rajesh Pahwa, MD, Laverne and Joyce Rider Professor of Neurology, Director, Parkinson's Disease and Movement Disorder Center, University of Kansas Medical Center, Kansas City, USA; Kelly E. Lyons, PhD, Research Professor of Neurology, Director of Research and Education, Parkinson's Disease and Movement Disorder Center, University of Kansas Medical Center, Kansas City, Kansas, USA. Edition: Fifth edition. Published/Produced: Boca Raton, FL: CRC Press, Taylor & Francis Group, [2013] ©2013 Description: xiv, 605 pages: illustrations; 24 cm ISBN: 9781841849089 (hardcover) 1841849081 (hardcover) LC classification: RC382 .H36 2013 Related names: Pahwa, Rajesh, editor of compilation. Lyons, Kelly E., editor of compilation. Contents: Early iconography of Parkinson's disease -- Epidemiology -- Differential diagnosis -- Pathophysiology and clinical assessment -- Premotor symptoms -- Autonomic dysfunction and management -- Sleep dysfunction -- Neuropsychological aspects -- Management of anxiety and depression -- Management of psychosis and dementia -- Neuroimaging -- Neuropathology of parkinsonism -- Neurophysiology -- Animal models of Parkinson's disease and related disorders -- Genetics -- Enviornmental risk factors -- Disease modification -- Amantadine and anticholonergics -- Levodopa -- dopamine agonists -- Monamine oxidase inhibitors -- Catechol-O-methyltransferase inhibitors -- Investigational pharmacological treatments -- Deep brain stimulation -- Investigational surgical therapies -- Physical and occupational therapy -- Voice, speech, and swallowing disorders -- Complementary and alternative medicine in Parkinson's diease. Subjects: Parkinson's disease--Handbooks, manuals, etc. Parkinson Disease. Notes: Includes bibliographical references and index.

Hankey's clinical neurology LCCN: 2014395481 Uniform title: Clinical neurology (Hankey) Main title: Hankey's clinical neurology / editors, Philip B. Gorelick, MD, MPH, FACP, FAHA, FAAN, FANA, Medical Director, Mercy Health Hauenstein Neuroscience Center at Saint Mary's, Professor, Translational Science & Molecular Medicine, Michigan State University College of Human Medicine, Grand Rapids, Michigan, USA, Fernando D. Testai, MD, PhD, FAHA, Assistant Professor in Neurology, University of Illinois College Medicine at Chicago, Chicago, Illinois, USA, Graeme J. Hankey, MBBS, MD, FRACP, FRCP, FRCPE, Winthrop Professor of Neurology, School of Medicine and Pharmacology, The University of Western Australia, Consultant Neurologist, Department of Neurology, Sir Charles Gairdner Hospital, Perth, Australia, Joanna M. Wardlaw, MBChB, MRCP, DMRD, FRCR, MD, FRCP, FMedSc, Professor of Applied Neuroimaging, Division of Clinical Neurosciences, University of Edinburgh, Western General Hospital, Edinburgh, UK.

Edition: Second edition. Published/Created: Boca Raton: CRC Press/Taylor & Francis Group, [2014] Description: 975 pages: illustrations (chiefly color); 27 cm ISBN: 9781840761931 (hardback: acid-free paper) 1840761938 (hardback: acid-free paper) LC classification: RC346 .H2356 2014 Portion of title: Clinical neurology Related names: Gorelick, Philip B. Testai, Fernando D. Hankey, Graeme J. Wardlaw, Joanna M. Contents: Machine generated contents note: ch. 1 Neurologic diagnosis / Robert Edis -- Introduction -- The diagnostic process in neurology -- Neurologic examination -- Lumbar puncture and CSF examination / John Dunne -- Neurophysiologic examination / William McAuliffe -- Imaging the brain and spine -- ch. 2 Disorders of consciousness / Venkatesh Aiyagari -- Impaired consciousness -- Brain death -- Persistent/permanent vegetative state -- Minimally conscious state -- Locked-in syndrome -- Syncope -- Hypoxic--ischemic encephalopathy -- Central pontine myelinolysis -- ch. 3 Epilepsy / Andres M. Kanner -- Definition -- Epidemiology -- Pathophysiology -- Classification -- Clinical features -- Differential diagnosis -- Investigation and diagnosis -- Treatment -- ch. 4 Headache / Peter J. Goadsby -- Headache -- Migraine -- Tension-type headache -- Cluster headache -- ch. 5 Vertigo / Jorge Kattah -- Introduction -- Specific syndromes -- ch. 6 Hyperkinetic movement disorders / Philip Thompson -- Introduction -- Dystonia -- Chorea -- Tremor -- Myoclonus -- Tics -- Stereotypies -- Dyskinesias -- Drug-induced movement disorders -- Psychogenic movement disorders -- ch. 7 Developmental diseases of the nervous system / James H. Tonsgard -- Introduction -- Embryonic development of the nervous system -- Developmental malformations of the nervous system -- Defects in neural tube formation -- Defects in hindbrain development -- Defects in forebrain and cerebral development -- Neurocutaneous disorders -- Neurofibromatosis Type 1 -- Neurofibromatosis Type 2 -- Tuberous sclerosis -- Sturge--Weber syndrome -- Hereditary hemorrhagic telangiectasia (Osler--Rendu--Weber syndrome) -- Linear nevus sebaceous syndrome -- Cowden's syndrome and Lhermitte--Duclos disease -- von Hippel--Lindau disease -- Incontinentia pigmenti -- Hypomelanosis of Ito -- ch. 8 Hereditary and metabolic diseases of the central nervous system in adults / Alma R. Bicknese -- Introduction -- Metabolic and degenerative diseases in adults -- Huntington's disease -- Cerebral autosomal dominant arteriopathy with subcortical infarcts and leukoencephalopathy -- Fragile X-associated tremor/ataxia syndrome -- X-linked adrenoleukodystrophy -- Pantothenate kinase-associated neurodegeneration -- Inherited diseases with prominent visceral and neurologic findings -- Wilson's disease -- Acute intermittent porphyria -- Disorders of amino acid metabolism -- Homocystinuria -- Inclusion body disorders -- Lafora body disease -- Adult neuronal ceroid lipofuscinoses -- Late-onset lysosomal storage diseases -- Late-onset GM2 gangliosidosis -- Late-onset metachromatic leukodystrophy -- Fabry's disease -- Late-onset Krabbe disease -- Niemann--Pick Type C -- Mitochondrial disorders -- Diseases of mitochondrial DNA -- ch. 9 Trauma of the brain and spinal cord / Prasad S.S.V. Vannemreddy -- Introduction -- Head injury -- Concussion -- Spinal cord injury -- ch. 10 Stroke and transient ischemic attacks of the brain and eye / Graeme J. Hankey -- Introduction -- Epidemiology -- Pathology and etiology -- Risk factors -- Clinical assessment -- Investigations -- Diagnosis -- Prognosis -- Treatment -- ch. 11 Infections of the central nervous system / James L. Cook -- Acute bacterial meningitis -- Brain abscess -- Neurosyphilis -- Lyme disease -- Tuberculosis (TB) -- Botulism -- Tetanus -- Aseptic meningitis -- Viral encephalitis -- Rabies -- Poliomyelitis -- Progressive multifocal leukoencephalopathy (PML) -- Cryptococcosis -- Coccidioidomycosis -- Toxoplasmosis -- Neurocysticercosis -- Eosinophilic meningitis -- Creutzfeldt--Jakob disease (CJD) -- ch. 12 Inflammatory disorders of the nervous system / Neil Scolding -- Acute disseminated encephalomyelitis (post-infectious encephalomyelitis) -- Multiple sclerosis (MS) -- Neurosarcoidosis -- Cavernous sinus syndrome -- ch. 13 Tumors of the nervous system / Robert P. Dinapoli -- Neoplasia -- Gliomas -- Meningioma -- Craniopharyngioma -- Pituitary tumors -- Vestibular schwannoma (acoustic neuroma) -- Primary central nervous system lymphoma -- Germ cell tumors of the CNS -- von Hippel--Lindau disease -- Metastases to the CNS -- Paraneoplastic neurologic disease -- ch. 14 Degenerative diseases of the nervous system / James A. Mastrianni -- Dementia -- Alzheimer's disease (AD) -- Frontotemporal dementia (FTD) -- Dementia with Lewy bodies (DLB) -- Vascular dementia -- Prion diseases -- Normal pressure hydrocephalus / Kathleen M. Shannon -- Parkinson's disease and parkinsonian disorders -- Introduction -- Primary (idiopathic) parkinsonism: Parkinson's disease -- Multisystem degenerations (Parkinsonism plus' or atypical parkinsonism) -- Heredodegenerative and secondary parkinsonism / Peter Todd -- Hereditary ataxias -- Introduction -- Congenital ataxias -- Autosomal dominant cerebellar ataxias -- Autosomal recessive cerebellar ataxias -- X-linked causes of ataxia -- ch. 15 Acquired metabolic diseases of the nervous system / Fernando D. Testai -- Thiamine deficiency: Wernick--Korsakoff syndrome -- Vitamin B12 deficiency -- Vitamin E deficiency -- Niacin (nicotinic acid) deficiency -- Marchiafava--Bignami disease -- Hepatic encephalopathy -- Uremic encephalopathy -- Posterior reversible encephalopathy syndrome -- ch. 16 Disorders of circulation of the cerebrospinal fluid / Edward A. Michals -- Introduction -- Aqueductal stenosis with hydrocephalus -- Communicating hydrocepahalus -- Normal pressure hydrocephalus -- Chiari malformation -- Syringomyelia (syringohydromyelia) -- Idiopathic intracranial hypertension (pseudotumor cerebri) -- Intracranial hypotension syndrome -- ch. 17 Cranial neuropathies I, V, and VII--XII / Helene Rubeiz -- Olfactory nerve neuropathy (cranial nerve I) -- Trigeminal nerve neuropathy (cranial nerve V) -- Selected conditions affecting the trigeminal nerve -- Facial nerve neuropathy (cranial nerve VII) -- Selected conditions affecting the facial nerve -- Vestibulo-cochlear nerve neuropathy (cranial nerve VIII) -- Glossopharyngeal nerve neuropathy (cranial nerve IX) -- Selected conditions affecting the glossopharyngeal nerve -- Vagus nerve neuropathy (cranial nerve X) -- Spinal accessory nerve neuropathy (cranial nerve XI) -- Hypoglossal nerve neuropathy (cranial nerve XII) -- ch. 18 Cranial neuropathies II, III, IV, and VI / Molly E. Gilbert -- Optic nerve neuropathy (cranial nerve II) -- Cranial nerve III, IV, and VI palsies -- ch. 19 Spinal cord disease / Octavia Kincaid -- Introduction to myelopathy --

Extramedullar spinal cord lesions (extrinsic myelopathy) -- Intramedullary spinal cord lesions (intrinsic myelopathy) -- Inflammatory myelopathy (e.g., myelitis) -- Infectious myelopathy -- Metabolic and toxic myelopathies -- Vascular myelopathies -- Structural myelopathies -- Hereditary myelopathies -- Spinal cord tumors -- Myelopathy associated with motor neuron disease -- ch. 20 Autonomic nervous system disorders / Judy Spies -- Autonomic neuropathy -- ch. 21 Diseases of the peripheral nerve and mononeuropathies / Andrea Swenson -- Peripheral neuropathy -- Diabetic neuropathy -- Toxic neuropathy -- Nutrition-related neuropathy -- Neuropathy in systemic disease -- Guillain--Barre syndrome (GBS)/Acute inflammatory demyelinating polyradiculoneuropathy (AIDP) -- Chronic acquired demyelinating polyneuropathy -- Vasculitic neuropathy -- Immune-mediated brachial plexus neuropathy (IBPN) -- Infectious neuropathy -- Hereditary motor and sensory neuropathy (Charcot--Marie--Tooth disease) -- Syndromic hereditary peripheral neuropathies -- Mononeuropathies -- Upper extremity neuropathy -- Lower extremity neuropathy -- ch. 22 Neuromuscular junction disorders / Julie Rowin -- Myasthenia gravis -- Congenital myasthenic syndromes -- Lambert--Eaton myasthenic syndrome -- Botulism -- ch. 23 Muscle disorders / Betty Soliven -- Introduction -- Myopathy -- Inflammatory myopathy -- Critical illness myopathy -- Endocrine and metabolic myopathies -- Muscular dystrophies -- Muscle channelopathies (disorders of membrane excitability) -- ch. 24 Sleep disorders / Michael Kohrman -- Introduction -- Normal sleep -- Commonly performed sleep tests -- Insomnias -- Hypersomnias of central origin -- Sleep-related movement disorders -- Sleep-related breathing disorders -- Circadian rhythm sleep disorders -- Parasomnias -- Conclusion. Subjects: Neurology. Nervous system--Diseases. Notes: Includes bibliographical references and index.

Marsden's book of movement disorders LCCN: 2012471553 Main title: Marsden's book of movement disorders / Ivan Donaldson ... [et al.]. Published/Created: Oxford: Oxford University Press, 2012. Description: xiv, 1497 p.: ill., ports.; 28 cm. ISBN:

9780192619112 (alk. paper) 019261911X (alk. paper) LC classification: RC376.5 .M37 2012 Variant title: Book of movement disorders Portion of title: Movement disorders Related names: Marsden, C. David. Donaldson, Ivan. Contents: Sect. 1. Structure and function of the basal ganglia. Anatomy functions of the basal ganglia -- Sect. 2. Clinical approach to movement disorders. Clinical assessment -- Investigation -- Sect. 3. Akinetic-rigid syndromes. Introduction -- Sect. 3A. Idiopathic/primary syndromes. Parkinson's disease -- Multiple system atrophy -- Progressive supranuclear palsy (or Steele-Richardson-Olszewski disease) -- Corticobasal degeneration -- Parkinsonian-dementia syndromes -- Sect. 3B. Symptomatic parkinsonian syndromes inherited. Wilson's disease -- Pantothenate kinase-associated neurodegeneration (PKAN), previously also known as Hallervorden-Spatz disease -- Sect. 3C. Symptomatic parkinsonian syndromes acquired. Postencephalic parkinsonism -- Drug-induced parkinsonism and the neuroleptic malginant syndrome -- Basal ganglia calcification -- Other acquired symptomatic parkinsonian syndromes -- Sect. 4. Tremor. Introduction. Physiological and exaggerated or enhanced physiological tremor -- Classical essential tremor -- Isolated site-specific or task-specific tremors -- Symptomatic tremors -- Sect. 5. Chorea. Introduction. Sect. 5A. Idiopathic choreic syndromes. Huntington's disease -- Other idiopathic choreic syndromes -- Sect. 5B. Symptomatic choreic syndromes. Sydenham's chorea -- Spontaneous oro-facial chorea and tardive dyskinesia -- Other symptomatic (secondary) choreic syndromes -- Ballism -- Sect. 6. Tics. Introduction. Sect. 6A. Idiopathic (primary) tic syndromes. Simple tics -- Gilles de la Tourette's syndrome -- Symptomatic (secondary) tic syndromes -- Sect. 7. Myoclonus. Focal myoclonus -- Epileptic myoclonus -- Brainstem myoclonus and startle syndromes -- Specific myoclonic syndromes -- Other specific causes of symptomatic generalized myoclonus -- Essential myoclonus -- Sect. 8. Dystonia. Introduction. Sect. 8A. Primary (idiopathic) dystonic syndromes. Generalized primary dystonia -- Other primary dystonias (dystonia-plus syndromes) -- Idiopathic (primary) cranial dystonias -- Spasmodic torticollis -- Writer's and craft cramps --

Sect. 8B. Secondary (symptomatic) dystonic syndromes. Lesch-Nyhan syndrome -- Other inherited secondary (symptomatic) dystonias -- Cerebral palsy -- Other acquired secondary (symptomatic) dystonic syndromes -- Sect. 9. Syndromes of continuous muscle fibre activity. Introduction. Stiff man syndromes -- Neuromyotonic syndromes -- Sect. 10. Restlessness. Introduction. Akathisia -- Restless legs syndrome -- Painful legs and moving toes -- Sect. 11. Episodic movement disorders. Introduction. Paroxysmal choreic, athetotic, or dystonic attacks -- Tonic attacks -- Intermittent ataxias -- Sect. 12. Miscellaneous movement disorders. Miscellaneous movement disorders. Subjects: Movement disorders. Movement Disorders. Notes: Includes bibliographical references and index.

Neurogenetics: a guide for clinicians LCCN: 2011026299 Main title: Neurogenetics: a guide for clinicians / edited by Nicholas W. Wood. Published/Created: Cambridge: Cambridge University Press, 2012. Description: vii, 241 p.: ill.; 25 cm. ISBN: 9780521543729 (pbk.) LC classification: RC346.4 .N482 2012 Related names: Wood, N. W. (Nicholas W.) Summary: "Progress in genetic knowledge is profoundly affecting medical practice, and no clinical specialty has more diseases associated with genetic mutations than neurology. As a more complete picture of the genes which give rise to neurological disease is obtained, trainee and practising neurologists need a guide to basic principles and the more important clinical entities with a genetic component. It is against this background that Neurogenetics: A Guide for Clinicians has been written. The book opens with coverage of genetic testing and counselling. Subsequent chapters discuss genetic factors for all the major neurological diseases, including epilepsy, Alzheimer's disease, Parkinsonism and muscular dystrophies. No book in this field can hope to be fully up to date with the latest research; rather this work provides a framework on which to add new genetic discoveries. Neurogenetics: A Guide for Clinicians provides a synoptic overview for neurologists, medical geneticists and scientists working in the field"--Provided by publisher. Contents: Machine generated contents note: Preface; 1. The human genome project -

what it really means and where next? / Sonia Gandhi and Nicholas Wood; 2. Genetic counselling and genetic testing for neurogenetic disorders / David Craufurd and Peter S. Harper; 3. Alzheimer's disease and related dementias / John Hardy; 4. The epilepsies / Mark Gardiner; 5. The ataxias / S. H. Subramony; 6. Huntington's disease / Sarah J. Tabrizi and Edward J. Wild; 7. Parkinsonism / Vincenzo Bonifati; 8. Prion diseases / Simon Mead and John Collinge; 9. Channelopathies / Michael G. Hanna and Dimitri M. Kullmann; 10. Amyotrophic lateral sclerosis and other disorders of the lower motor neuron / Christopher E. Shaw ... [et sl.]; 11. The muscular dystrophies / Kate Bushby and Una Sheerin; 12. Charcot-Marie-Tooth diseases / Odile Dubourg, Alexis Brice, and Eric LeGuern; 13. Mitochondrial disorders / Robert McFarland ... [et al.]; 14. The neurofibromatoses and related disorders / Rosalie E. Ferner; 15. The future of neurogenetics / Thomas D. Bird. Subjects: Nervous system--Diseases--Genetic aspects. Neurogenetics. Nervous System Diseases--genetics. Genetic Diseases, Inborn--etiology. Genetic Testing. Notes: Includes bibliographical references and index.

Neurology for the hospitalist: a practical approach LCCN: 2013026662 Personal name: Likosky, David J., author. Main title: Neurology for the hospitalist: a practical approach / David Likosky, MD, SFHM, EvergreenHealth Medical Center, S. Andrew Josephson, MD, University of California San Francisco, Michael J. Pistoria, DO, FACP, SFHM, Lehigh Valley Health Network, W. David Freeman, MD, Mayo Clinic. Published/Produced: Oxford; New York: Oxford University Press, [2014] Description: ix, 189 pages: illustrations; 21 cm ISBN: 9780199969630 (pbk.: acid-free paper) LC classification: RC348 .L56 2014 Related names: Josephson, Scott Andrew, author. Pistoria, Michael Joseph, author. Freeman, William D., author. Contents: Overview of neuroanatomy -- History and physical -- Stroke overview/pathophysiology -- TIA evaluation -- Ischemic stroke -- Hemorrhagic stroke -- Venous sinus thrombosis -- Elevated intracranial pressure -- CNS demyelinating disorders -- Meningitis and encephalitis -- Spinal epidural abscess -- Seizure

-- Status epilepticus -- Syncope -- Headache -- Delirium -- Dementia -- Coma and brain death -- Approach to and management of the patient with weakness -- Parkinsons disease/Parkinsonism -- Dystonic reactions -- Neoplastic disorders -- Paraneoplastic neurologic disorders -- Visual disturbances -- Vertigo and dizziness -- Other spinal cord processes. Subjects: Central Nervous System Diseases--diagnosis--Handbooks. Hospitalists--Handbooks. Neurologic Examination--Handbooks. Neurologic Manifestations--Handbooks. Notes: Includes index.

Pharmacology: a nursing process approach LCCN: 2011006456 Personal name: Kee, Joyce LeFever. Main title: Pharmacology: a nursing process approach / Joyce LeFever Kee, Evelyn R. Hayes, Linda E. McCuistion. Edition: 7th ed. Published/Created: St. Louis, MO: Elsevier Saunders, c2012. Description: xxiv, 978 p.: col. ill.; 28 cm. ISBN: 9781437717112 (pbk.: alk. paper) 143771711X (pbk.: alk. paper) LC classification: RM301 .K44 2012 Related names: Hayes, Evelyn R. McCuistion, Linda E. Contents: Drug action: pharmaceutic, pharmacokinetic and pharmacodynamic phases -- Nursing process and client teaching -- Medication safety -- Medication administration -- Medications and calculations -- The drug approval process -- Cultural and pharmacogenetic considerations -- Drug interactions and over-the-counter drugs -- Drugs of abuse -- Herbal therapy with nursing implications -- Pediatric pharmacology -- Geriatric pharmacology -- Medication administration in community settings -- The role of the nurse in drug research -- Vitamin and mineral replacement -- Fluid and electrolyte replacement -- Nutritional support -- Adrenergic agonists and adrenergic blockers -- Cholinergic agonists and anticholinergics -- Central nervous system stimulants -- Central nervous system depressants -- Anticonvulsants -- Drugs for neurologic disorders: Parkinsonism and Alzheimer's Disease -- Drugs for neuromuscular disorders: myasthenia gravis, multiple sclerosis, and muscle spasms -- Antiinflammatory drugs -- Nonopioid and opioid analgesics -- Antipsychotics and anxiolytics -- Antidepressants and mood stabilizers -- Penicillins and cephalosporins -- Macrolides, tetracyclines, aminoglycosides, and fluoroquinolones -- Sulfonamides -- Antituberculars, antifungals, peptides, and metronidazole -- Antivirals, antimalarials, and anthelmintics -- Drugs for urinary tract disorders -- HIV- and AIDS-related drugs -- Vaccines -- Anticancer drugs -- Targeted therapies to treat cancer -- Biologic response modifiers -- Drugs for upper respiratory disorders -- Drugs for lower respiratory disorders -- Cardiac glycosides, antianginals, and antidysrhythmics -- Diuretics -- Antihypertensives -- Anticoagulants, antiplatelets, and thrombolytics -- Antihyperlipidemics and peripheral vasodilators -- Drugs for gastrointestinal tract disorders -- Antiulcer drugs -- Drugs for eye and ear disorders -- Drugs for dermatologic disorders -- Endocrine drugs: pituitary, thyroid, parathyroid, and adrenal disorders -- Antidiabetes -- Female reproductive cycle I: pregnancy and preterm labor drugs -- Female reproductive cycle II: labor, delivery, and preterm neonatal drugs -- Postpartum and newborn drugs -- Drugs for women's reproductive health and menopause -- Drugs for men's health and reproductive disorders -- Drugs for disorders in women's health, infertility, and sexually transmitted infections -- Adult and pediatric emergency drugs. Subjects: Pharmacology. Nursing. Pharmacological Phenomena--Nurses' Instruction. Drug Therapy--Nurses' Instruction. Pharmaceutical Preparations--Nurses' Instruction. Notes: Includes bibliographical references and index.

Sleep disorders in neurology LCCN: 2011028725 Main title: Sleep disorders in neurology / Rosalia Silvestri, editor. Published/Created: Hauppauge, N.Y.: Nova Science Publishers, c2012. Description: vi, 391 p.: ill.; 27 cm. ISBN: 9781614705741 (hardcover) LC classification: RC547 .S526 2012 Related names: Silvestri, Rosalia. Contents: Idiopathic insomnia and fatal familial insomnia / F. Provini -- Narcolepsy / G. Mayer -- CNS hypersomnia / M. Billiard -- Kleine levin and other recurrent cyclic hypersomnias / M. Savarese -- EDS in neurological disorders / E. Bonanni ... [et al.] -- Disorders of arousal / R. Silvestri -- Hypnagogic hallucinations and sleep paralysis / G.L. Gigli -- Nightmares / A. Zadra -- REM behavior disorder / M.L. Fantini -- Periodic leg movement disorder / R. Ferri, L. Novelli, O. Bruni -- Restless leg syndrome / A. Walters -- Bruxism and catathrenia / G. Plazzi, K.K. Moghadam -- Sleep rhythmic related movement disorder / R. Manni -- Epilepsy and sleep / L. Nobili, G. Didato -- Headache and sleep / P. Montagna -- Sleep disorders in multiple sclerosis and amyotrophic lateral sclerosis / M. Manconi -- Parkinsonism and related disorders and sleep / M. Seyffert, S. Chokroverty -- Dementia and sleep / R. Mutani, A. Cicolin -- OSAS in neurology / C. Guilleminault -- CSA and congenital hypoventilation syndrome / L. Ferini-Strambi -- Cerebro-vascular disorders and sleep / C. Bassetti -- CNS vasculitis and sleep disorders / A. Walters -- Sleep disorders in peripheral neuropathies / C. Gaig, A. Iranzo -- Sleep disorders in miastenia gravis and miopathies / G. Mennuni, G. Della Marca. Subjects: Sleep Disorders--etiology. Sleep Disorders--physiopathology. Nervous System Diseases--complications. Notes: Includes bibliographical references and index. Series: Sleep - physiology, functions, dreaming and disorders Neurology - laboratory and clinical research developments

Upwards: the story of my struggle with Parkinsonism LCCN: 2014434328 Personal name: Reinman, Shami, -2015 author. Main title: Upwards: the story of my struggle with Parkinsonism / Shami Reinman. Edition: First edition - first impression. Published/Produced: [Brooklyn, NY]: The Shaar Press, [2014] Brooklyn, N.Y.: Distributed by Mesorah Publications, LTD Description: 278 pages: illustrations; 23 cm ISBN: 9781422614792 1422614794 LC classification: RC382 .R45 2014 Subjects: Reinman, Shami, -2015 Parkinson's disease--Patients--New Jersey--Biography. Jewish women--New Jersey--Lakewood--Biography.

INDEX

D

E

I

J

K

L

M

N

O

P

Q

R

S